Self-assessment
Oral
Radiology

MW01596532

P G J Rout
BDS FDSRCS MDentSC DDRRCR

The University of Birmingham
Dental School
Birmingham
UK

R M Browne
BSc DDS PhD FDSRCS FRCPath

The University of Birmingham
Dental School
Birmingham
UK

M Mosby-Wolfe

London • Baltimore • Barcelona • Bogotá • Boston
Buenos Aires • Carlsbad, CA • Chicago • Madrid
Mexico City • Milan • Naples, FL • New York
Philadelphia • St. Louis • Seoul • Singapore
Sydney • Taipei • Tokyo • Toronto • Wiesbaden

Publisher: **Geoff Greenwood**

Development Editors: **Lucy Hamilton**

                      Simon Pritchard

Project Manager: **Leslie Sinoway**

Production: **Siobhan Egan**

Index: **A. Cottingham**

Design: **Lara Last**

Cover Design: **Greg Smith**

Copyright © 1997 Times Mirror International Publishers Limited

Published in 1997 by Mosby-Wolfe, an imprint of Times Mirror International Publishers Limited

Printed by Grafos, Barcelona, Spain.

ISBN 0 7234 2422 5

For full details of all Times Mirror International Publishers Limited titles, please write to Times Mirror International Publishers Limited, Lynton House, 7–12 Tavistock Square, London WC1H 9LB, UK.

A CIP catalogue record for this book is available from the British Library.

Preface

Radiograpy is probably the most common special investigation undertaken by dental practitioners. It is through this medium of dental radiographs, together with some of the newer imaging modalities, that this book provides a series of self-assessment tests. It illustrates conditions both common and unusual that may occur in clinical practice.

The book is aimed at the undergraduate, the recent graduate and the general dental practitioner undergoing further education. It covers topics from radiation protection and quality assurance to disorders that affect the teeth, jaws and related soft tissues. The answer section contains information to remind the reader of the conditions illustrated, together with some details on their management. The book is not intended to be comprehensive, nor is it designed to replace existing textbooks. However, it is hoped that it will be useful in the consolidation of knowledge and as preparation for an examination or test on diagnostic and radiographic problems.

The editors are grateful to all the contributors for supplying useful and interesting material. It is hoped that through the wide variety of examples illustrated and the information provided, this book will put the reader fully in the picture.

Acknowledgements

The editors wish to thank all the contributors, their secretaries and X-ray and photographic departments for the preparation of the material used in this book. The editors also acknowledge the assistance of Mrs Rita Cottrill and Mrs Glenda Knee with the preparation of the manuscript. The three radiographs illustrating questions 50, 86, 107 and 149, are reproduced from the *Atlas of Dental and Maxillofacial Radiology and Imaging,* Browne, Edmondson, Rout; Mosby-Wolfe, 1995.

Contributors

I L C Chapple, PhD, BDS, FDSRCPS.

H D Edmondson, MB, ChB, DDS, FDSRCS, MRCS, LRCP, DA.

P J Lumley, PhD, MDentSc, BDS, FDSFRPS.

L Shaw, BDS, PhD, LDS, FDSRCS.

A C C Shortall, DDS; BDS, FDSRCPS, FFDRCSI.

The University of Birmingham Dental School, Birmingham, UK

P N Hirschmann, MSc, FRDRCS, DDRRCR.

Leeds Dental Institute, Leeds, England

K Horner, MSc, BChD, FDSRCS, DDRRCR.

Turner Dental School, University of Manchester. UK

E J Whaites, MSc, BDS, FDSRCS, DDRRCR, LDSRCS.

J Brown, MSc, BDS, FDSRCPS, DDRRCR.

United Medical and Dental Schools University of London, UK

S N Rogers, BDS, MBChB, FDSRCS, FRCS.

Walton Hospital, Liverpool.

Annotation of the dentition

In this book we have used the Zsigmondy system for identifying the teeth. For those more familiar with the system recommended by the Fédération Dentaire Internationale (FDI), the two systems are compared below.

PERMANENT DENTITION

(18) (17) (16) (15) (14) (13) (12) (11)	(21) (22) (23) (24) (25) (26) (27) (28)
8 7 6 5 4 3 2 1	1 2 3 4 5 6 7 8
8 7 6 5 4 3 2 1	1 2 3 4 5 6 7 8
(48) (47) (46) (45) (44) (43) (42) (41)	(31) (32) (33) (34) (35) (36) (37) (38)

PRIMARY DENTITION

(55) (54) (53) (52) (51)	(61) (62) (63) (64) (65)
E D C B A	A B C D E
E D C B A	A B C D E
(85) (84) (83) (82) (81)	(71) (73) (73) (74) (75)

In the Zsigmondy system, each permanent tooth is represented by a single digit displayed in the appropriate quadrant of the mouth. Thus $\overline{6}$ designates the right mandibular permanent first molar. Above the maxillary teeth and below the mandibular teeth the corresponding codes (in brackets) are illustrated using the FDI system. This is a two-digit system in which there is an additional digit for each quadrant of the mouth. Thus 46 designates the right mandibular permanent first molar. The codes in both systems are modified as indicated for the primary dentition.

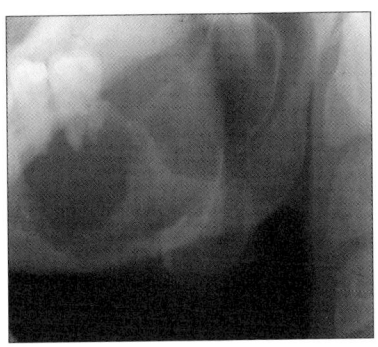

1 This 40-year-old complained of a painless swelling of his jaw and loosening of the lower posterior teeth.
(a) What is the radiographic view illustrated?
(b) What other radiographic investigations would you request and why?
(c) What are the main radiographic features of the lesion?
(d) What is the differential diagnosis?

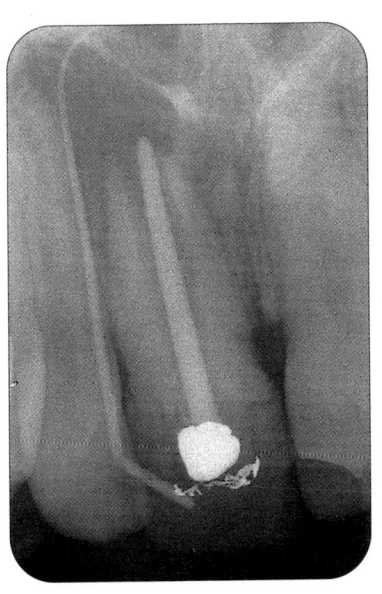

2 The patient, aged 28 years, complained of a discharge of pus through a sinus associated with the upper right central incisor tooth.
(a) What is the finer radiopaque line leading to the periapical radiolucency on this periapical radiograph?
(b) Describe the appearance of the root canal in the upper right central incisor and indicate the probable reason for its abnormal shape.
(c) What is the most likely diagnosis of the periapical radiolucency and how should it be managed?

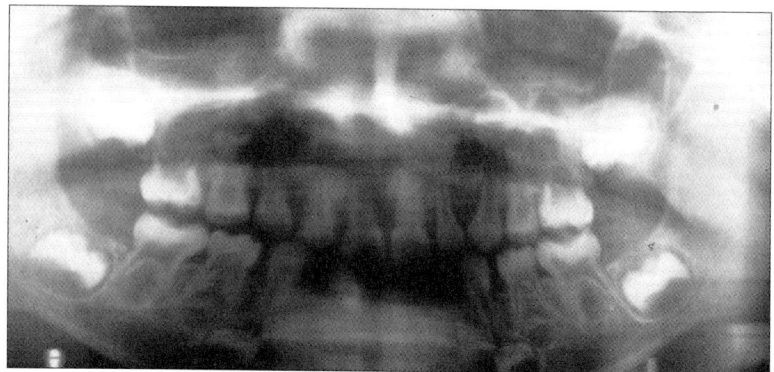

3 This dental panoramic tomograph of an 18-month-old boy shows premature loss of the primary lower incisor teeth, which had spontaneously exfoliated. He was subsequently found to have skeletal abnormalities similar to rickets.
(a) Besides the absence of the primary lower incisors, what other diagnostic features are present in and associated with the teeth?
(b) What is the underlying systemic condition?
(c) What other radiographic changes may be present in this condition?

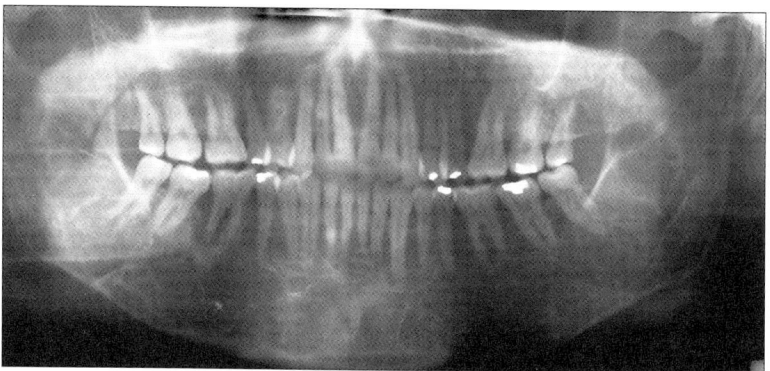

4 This 30-year-old complained of pain from his lower right first molar, which was diagnosed as a lateral periodontal abscess.
(a) What other abnormalities are present on this dental panoramic tomograph?
(b) What is the probable diagnosis?

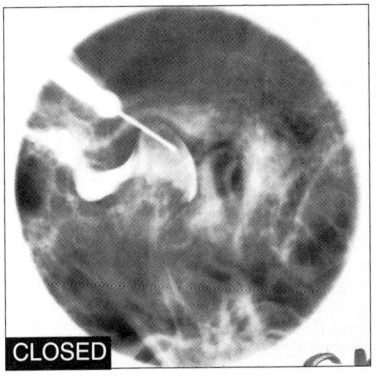

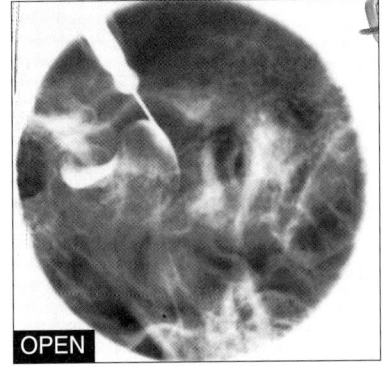

CLOSED

OPEN

5 The left temporomandibular joint (TMJ) is shown of a 24-year-old woman who complained of pain over that joint and limitation of mouth opening. The joint used to 'click' on opening and closing her mouth but when that recently stopped, her jaw opening became limited.
(a) What imaging technique is shown?
(b) What are the clinical indications for its use?
(c) What are the clinical contraindications to this technique?
(d) What is the diagnosis?

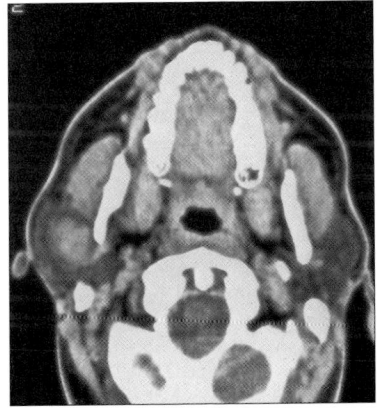

6 This 45-year-old has a persistent swelling of the right side of her face overlying the angle of the mandible, just in front of her ear.
(a) What type of image is illustrated?
(b) What abnormality is shown?
(c) What is the most likely diagnosis?
(d) What other imaging techniques may help in investigating such disorders?
(e) What is the treatment?

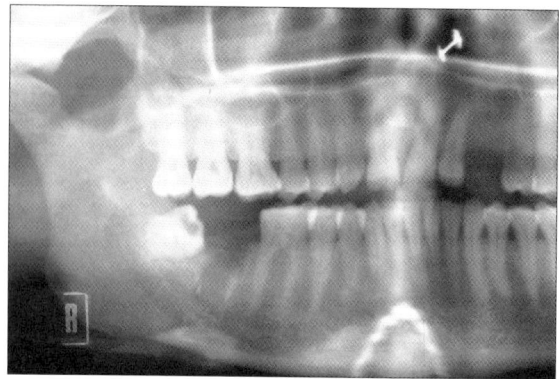

7 This patient, who had 7| extracted 8 days previously, complained of continuing discomfort.
(a) Describe the appearance of the tooth socket on this dental panoramic tomograph.
(b) What is the differential diagnosis of the discomfort?
(c) What radiological features may be of relevance in explaining why the tooth fractured during extraction?
(d) What additional radiograph(s) would be required in the surgical management of this patient?
(e) What is the foreign body in the region of the nose?

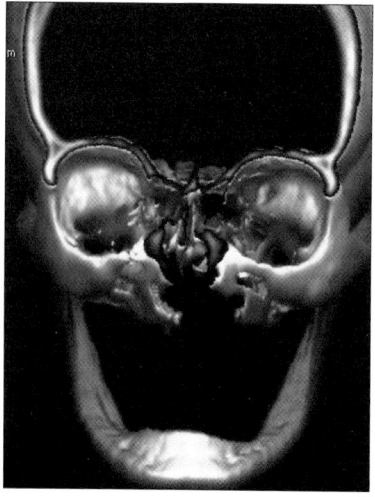

8 This 26-year-old patient suffered from severe hypodontia. The teeth had been extracted 10 years before.
(a) What type of image is illustrated?
(b) What are the main abnormalities?

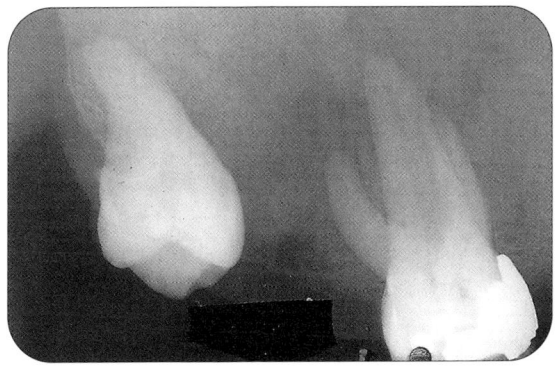

9 (a) What bony anomalies are evident on this periapical radiograph?
(b) List three conditions that can produce this radiographic appearance.
(c) What other investigations would you request to help in the diagnosis?

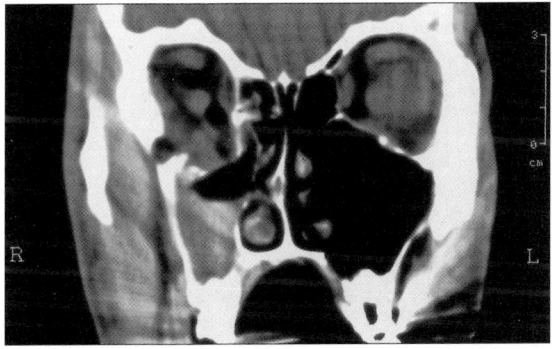

10 This patient received a blow to the face from a blunt object.
(a) Describe the abnormalities shown on this coronal computerized tomograph.
(b) What is the diagnosis?
(c) What are the cardinal signs and symptoms of this condition (other than pain and swelling)?
(d) What are the typical features that would be seen in an occipitomental radiograph of this condition?

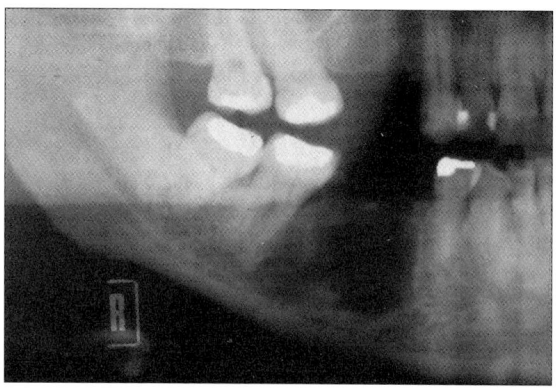

11 This dental panoramic tomograph was taken of a 30-year-old patient who complained of a swelling in the lower right first molar region.
(a) Describe the radiographic abnormality.
(b) Outline the differential diagnosis.

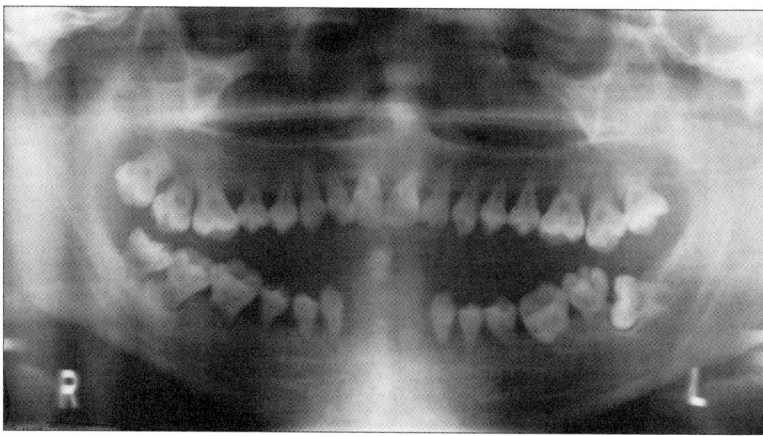

12 This 17-year-old male was concerned about his missing lower incisors. and reported that these teeth had fallen out approximately 10 years before.
(a) Describe the generalized abnormality of the teeth illustrated in this dental panoramic tomograph. What is the condition called?
(b) What disorders may be associated with this condition?

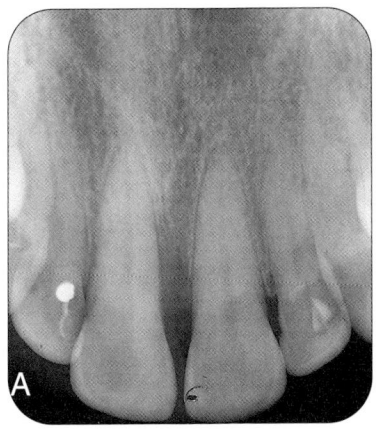
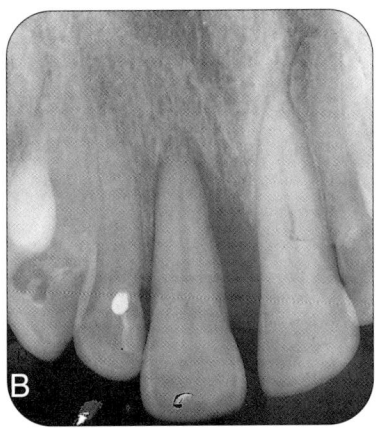

13 These two periapical radiographs are of the same patient, but Fig. 13A on the left was taken 9 months before that on the right. The patient was a 34-year-old woman with good oral hygiene.
(a) Describe the radiographic changes that have occurred during the 9 months.
(b) What is the diagnosis?
(c) What is the management of this case?

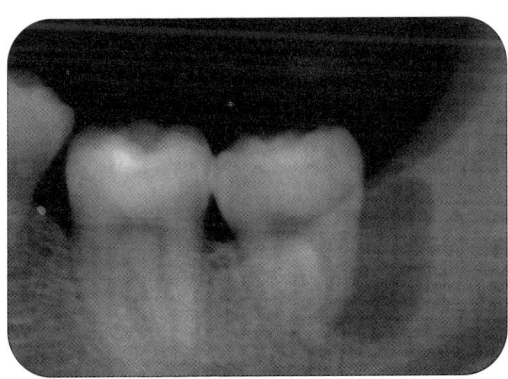

14 This patient gave a history of recurrent pericoronitis and buccal swelling associated with the partially erupted lower left wisdom tooth.
(a) Describe the main abnormality in this periapical radiograph.
(b) What is the most likely diagnosis?

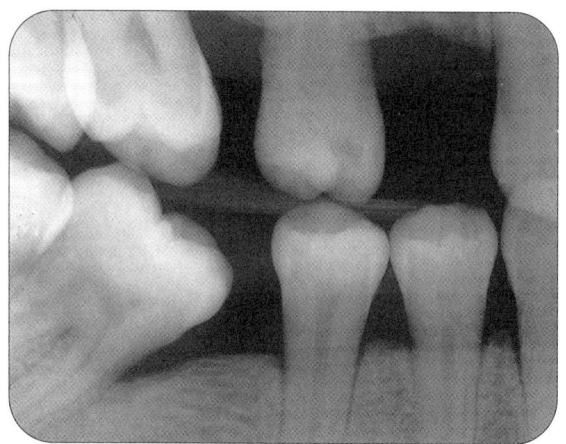

15 (a) What abnormalities are illustrated on this bitewing radiograph?
(b) What other radiographs are necessary?
(c) What is the probable cause of the abnormality present at the mesial aspect of $\overline{7|}$?

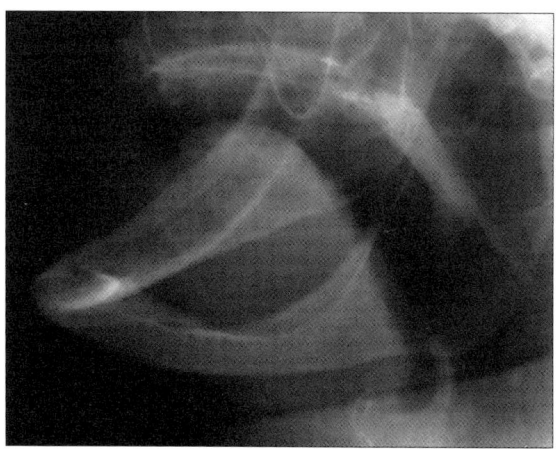

16 (a) Describe the appearance of the mandible on this oblique lateral radiograph.
(b) What is the most likely diagnosis?

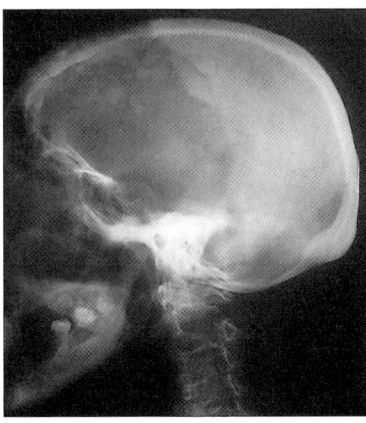

17 (a) What are the main radiographic changes on this true lateral skull radiograph?
(b) Of what orofacial abnormalities might this patient complain?
(c) From what condition is this elderly man suffering?

18 How would you explain to a patient the risk of radiation exposure associated with taking two bitewing radiographs?

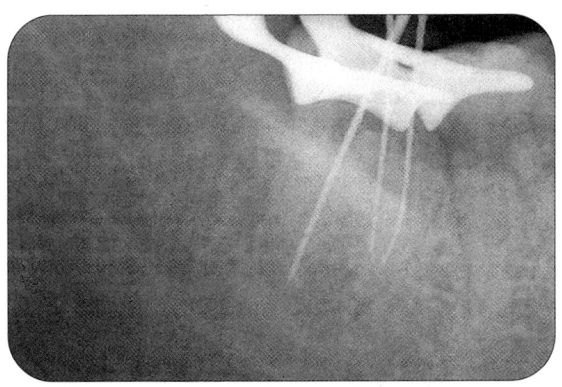

19 This periapical radiograph, taken to determine the working length of files, was exposed with the X-ray tube angled obliquely forwards relative to the tooth.
(a) Passing from the distal (left) to the mesial (right) aspect of the radiograph, which root canals contain files?
(b) What is the linear radiopaque object in the upper right-hand corner of the film?

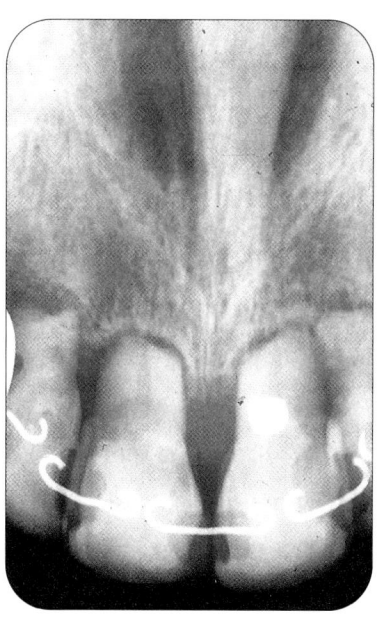

20 This 40-year-old woman has external root resorption affecting a number of her teeth, which have been splinted.
(a) Describe the abnormal features in this periapical radiograph.
(b) What are the possible causes of the root resorption?
(c) Outline the management.

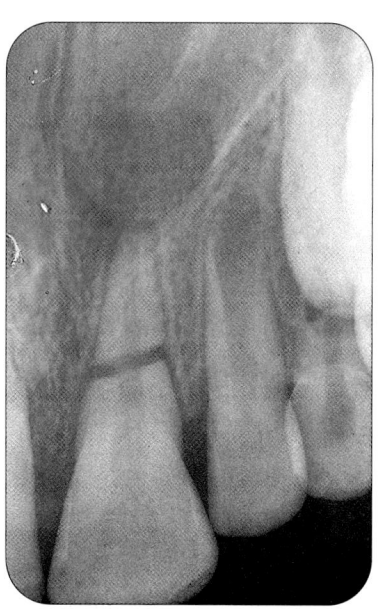

21 This patient received a blow to|1_ when he fell off his bicycle 6 months previously. The tooth exhibits grade one mobility and gives a negative response to thermal and electrical pulp stimulation.
(a) Estimate the age of the patient from the periapical radiograph.
(b) What is your diagnosis and what treatment would you recommend?

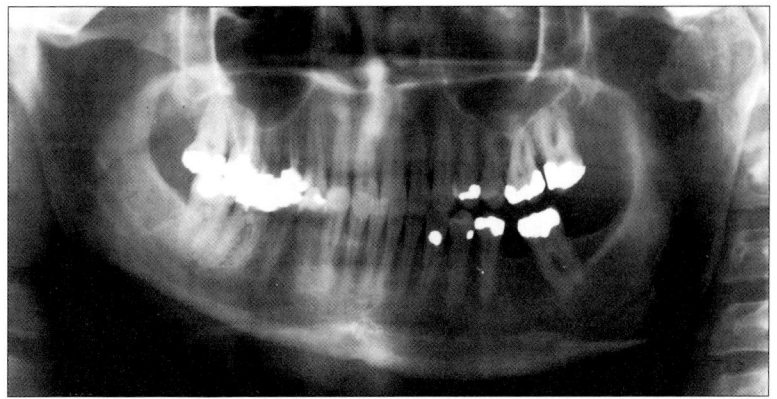

22 This 34-year-old patient gave a history of a slowly progressing facial asymmetry which began in adolescence.
(a) Describe the radiographic abnormalities in the dental panoramic tomograph.
(b) What is the differential diagnosis.

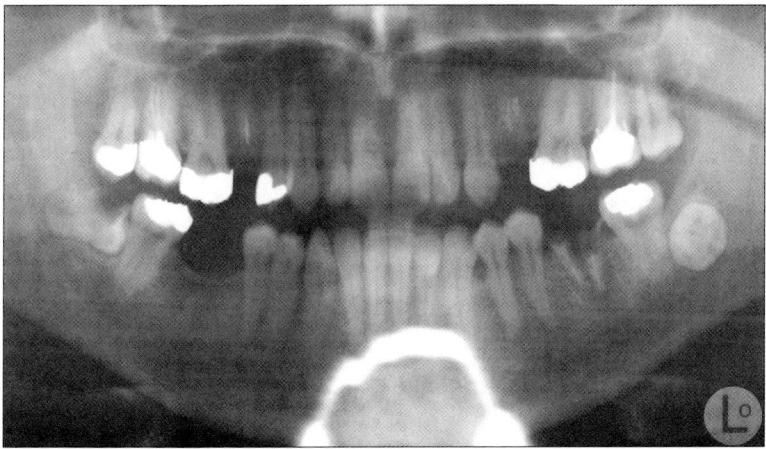

23 (a) Describe the main features in each quadrant of the dental panoramic tomograph.
(b) What is the likely dental history of this patient?
(c) What further radiographs may be helpful in the assessment of $\overline{8}$?
(d) What is the dense radiopaque structure overlying the mandible in the anterior region?

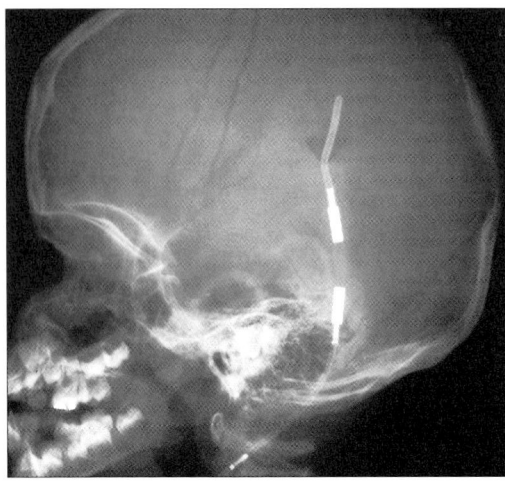

24 (a) What is the radiopaque structure shown on this lateral skull radiograph?
(b) Why was it inserted?
(c) What are the implications for the provision of dental care?

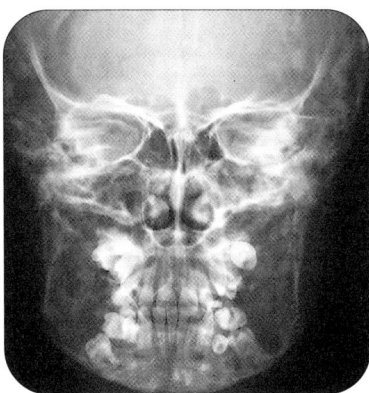

25 This 8-year-old girl complained of being bullied at school because she had a chubby face.
(a) What radiographic view is shown?
(b) How is it taken?
(c) What other radiographic views would you request?
(d) What are the main abnormalities shown in this radiograph?
(e) What is the most likely diagnosis?

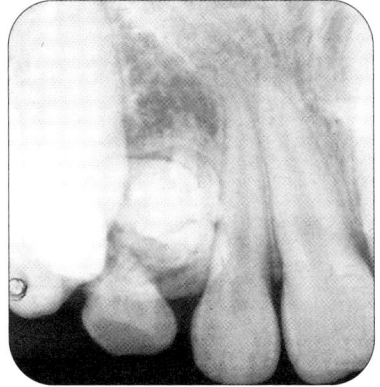

26 This periapical radiograph was taken to determine why 3| had failed to erupt.
(a) Describe the abnormality.
(b) What is the most likely diagnosis?
(c) What is the management?

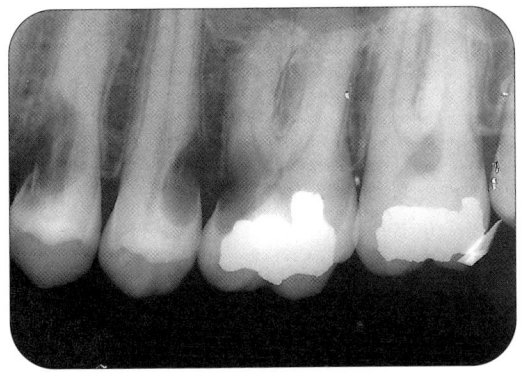

27 This is a periapical radiograph of a 21-year-old patient taken as part of a routine dental examination. The patient did not have any symptoms
(a) Describe the main radiographic abnormalities.
(b) What is the most likely diagnosis?

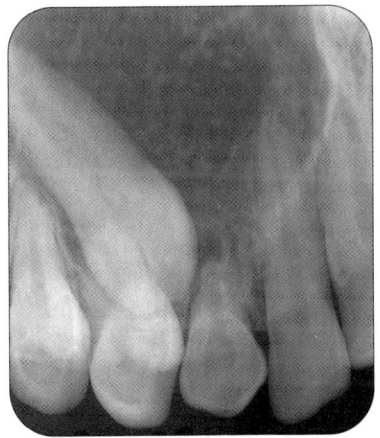

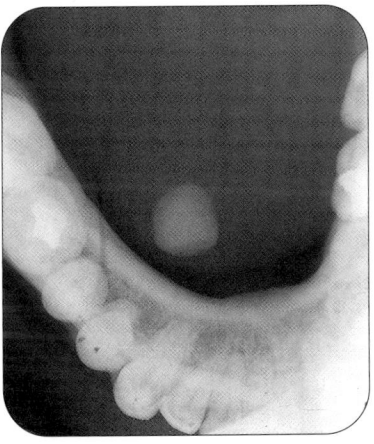

28 This 18-year-old woman asks your advice regarding increasing mobility of C|.
(a) Describe the abnormalities shown in this periapical radiograph.
(b) What is the most likely diagnosis?
(c) What is the management?

29 (a) What is the radiographic view illustrated?
(b) Describe the abnormality.
(c) What is the most likely diagnosis?
(d) What are the clinical features associated with this condition?

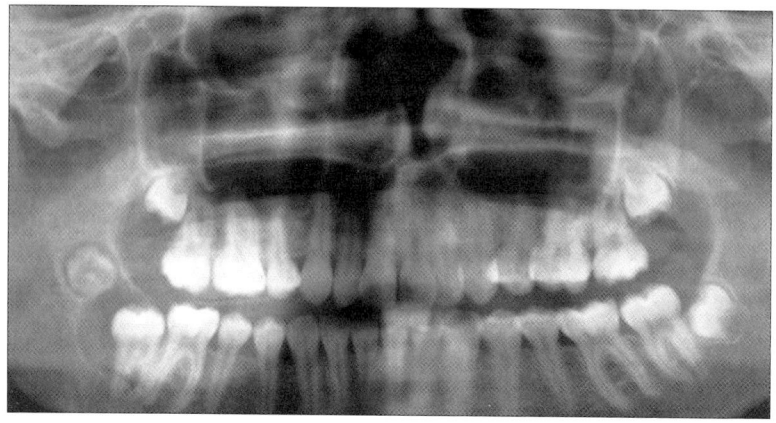

30 This 15-year-old boy attended because of pain in the right side of his jaw after a road traffic accident. It was a low velocity injury and he was wearing a seat belt. The right side of his face hit the steering wheel with minimal force.
(a) Describe the main abnormalities in this dental panoramic tomograph.
(b) What is the cause of the pain?

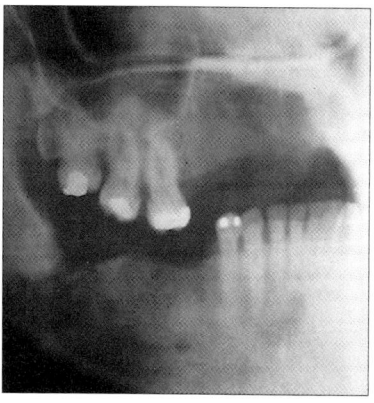

31 This 55-year-old woman complained of a dry mouth; a clinical examination revealed bilateral swelling of her parotid glands.
(a) What type of image is illustrated (see back cover for colour version)?
(b) How is the image formed?
(c) What is the main feature shown?
(d) What is the most likely diagnosis?
(e) What other features are likely to be present?
(f) Outline the management.

32 What procedures must be followed if a patient is overexposed accidentally during a dental X-ray examination?

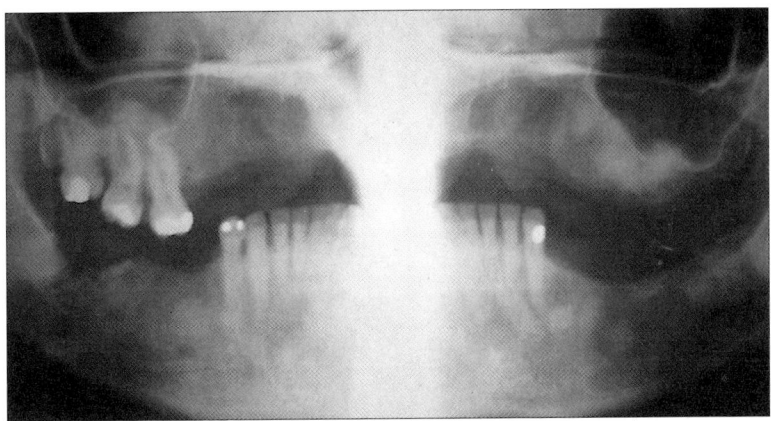

33 This 55-year-old African woman complained of pain following extraction of the lower right third molar 6 weeks previously.
(a) What condition is shown in this dental panoramic tomograph?
(b) Why is she experiencing pain from the extraction socket?

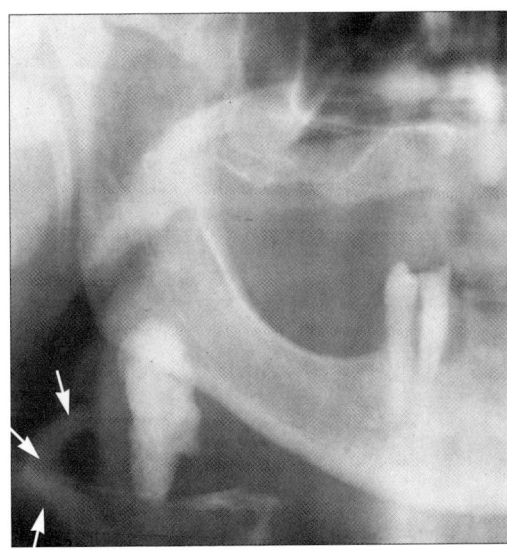

34 This dental panoramic tomograph was taken as part of the patient's assessment before the construction of dentures.
(a) Describe the abnormality shown in the region of the angle of the mandible.
(b) What is the most likely diagnosis?
(c) What is the radiopaque arcuate structure (arrowed)?

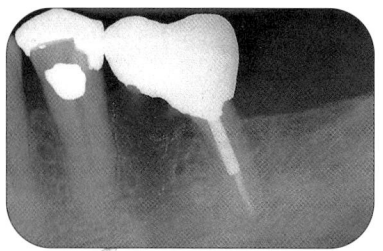

35 (a) From the evidence depicted on this periapical radiograph, what procedures have been undertaken on the lower left first molar?
(b) What complications may occur?

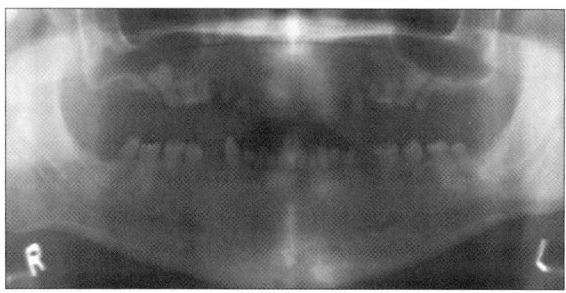

36 This 21-year-old patient was concerned about the appearance of his teeth, and complained of difficulty eating.
(a) Comment on the appearance of the roots and pulp chambers of the teeth in this dental panoramic tomograph.
(b) With what generalized pathological conditions may this appearance be associated?
(c) Outline the management.

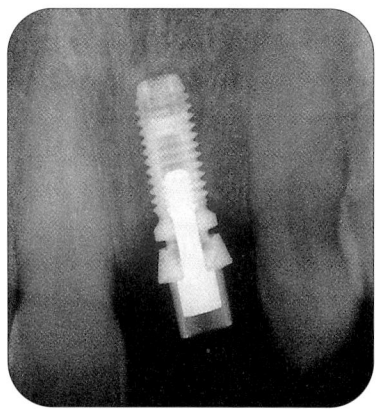

37 The radiograph, shows a 10 mm Brånemark implant inserted to replace|1. It was taken 4 months after implantation during the second operation after removal of the cover screw and insertion of the abutment.
(a) Has osseointegration taken place?
(b) Why should a radiograph be taken at this stage?
(c) What radiographic image should be obtained?
(d) Should the mucoperiosteal tissue be sutured immediately in view of the radiographic findings?

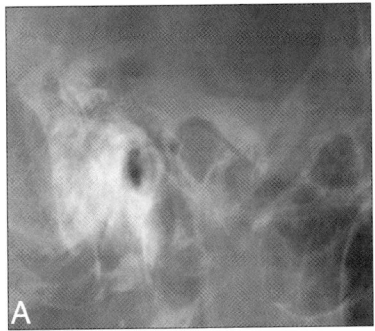
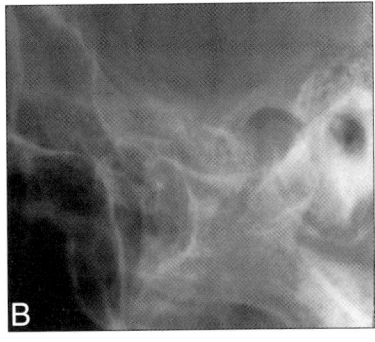

38 This 45-year-old woman complained of deviation of the jaw to the right on opening, limited opening, 'stiffness' and an ache in the region of the right TMJ, worsening as the day progressed. On examination there was tenderness over this joint and restricted movement, corresponding to the symptoms.

(a) What radiographs are illustrated?

(b) How are the X-ray beam, patient's head and film positioned relative to each other during the exposure?

(c) What normal features of the TMJ are shown by this projection?

(d) Describe the abnormalities in **38A** and **38B**.

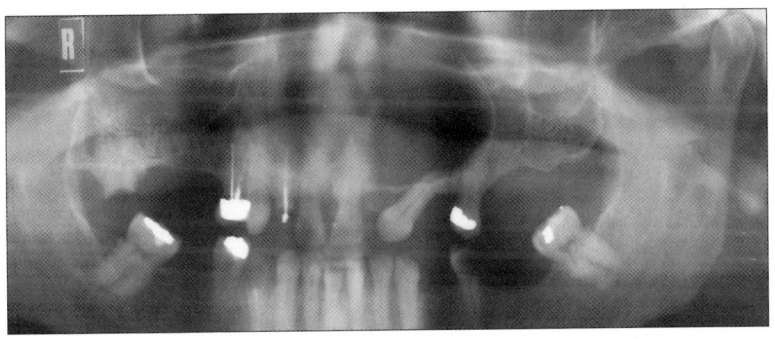

39 (a) What is the most obvious abnormality on this dental panoramic tomograph; describe its radiological features?

(b) What is the differential diagnosis and why?

(c) What might be the main clinical features?

(d) What clinical tests may aid the diagnosis?

(e) What additional radiographic views might be helpful before treatment?

(f) How might the lesion be treated and what radiological follow-up may be required?

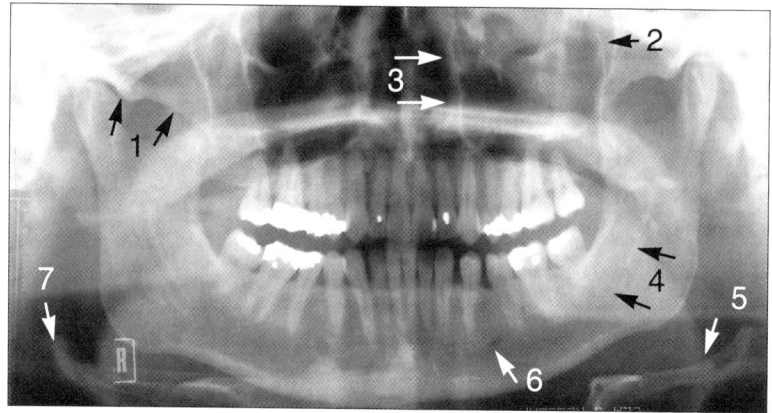

40 What are the anatomical structures **1–7** in this dental panoramic tomograph?

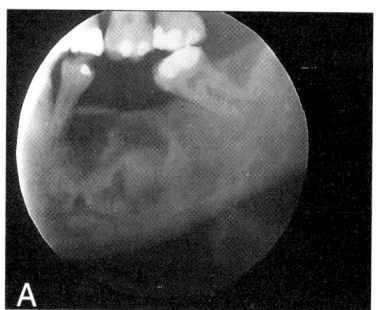

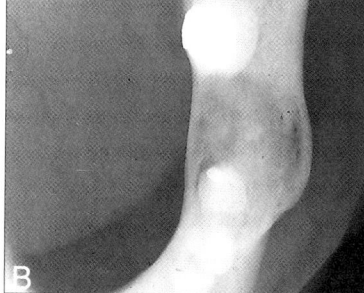

41 (a) What radiographic views of this 17-year-old are shown?
(b) What are the radiographic features of the lesion?
(c) What is the most likely diagnosis?

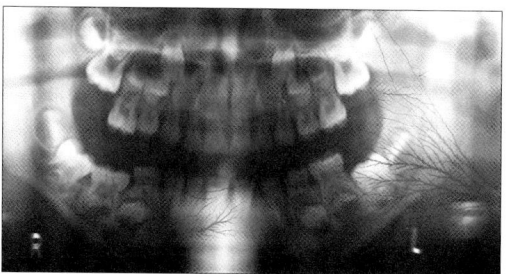

42 (a) What is the cause of the numerous branching radiolucent lines seen on this dental panoramic tomograph?
(b) How may this appearance be caused?

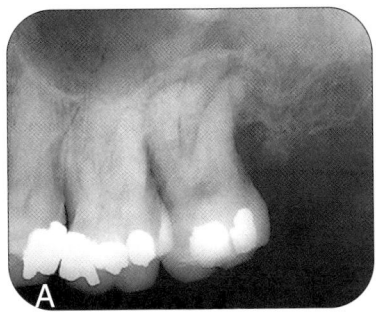

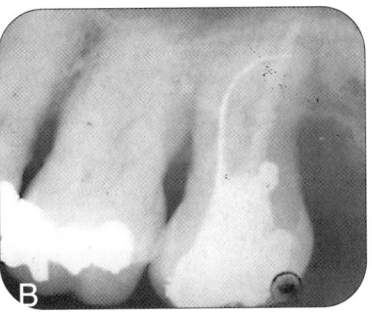

43 These periapical radiographs of $\underline{7|}$ were taken at the time of treatment (**43A**) and after 10 years (**43B**). What was the condition and what treatment was undertaken?

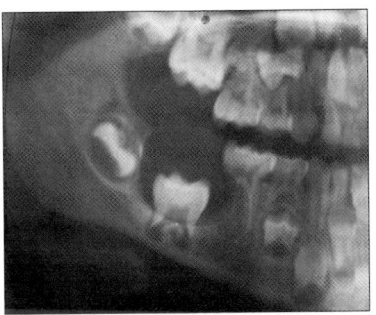

44 This dental panoramic tomograph of a 6-year-old was taken to investigate a swelling in the $\overline{6|}$ region.
(a) Describe the abnormality shown.
(b) What is the most likely diagnosis?
(c) How should it be managed?

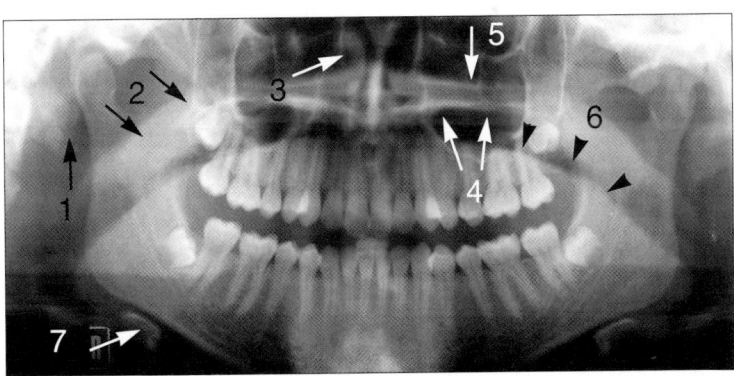

45 What are the anatomical structures identified by **1–7** in this dental panoramic tomograph?

46 You wish to take two bitewing radiographs to monitor caries progression, but the patient then tells you she is pregnant. Would you make any change to your radiographic procedure?

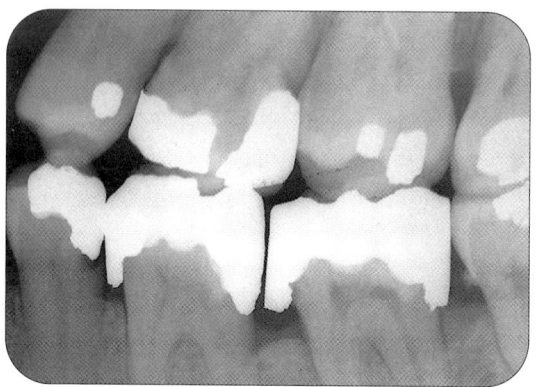

47 The amalgam restorations $\overline{67}$ shown in this bitewing radiograph have been in place for 5 years and have not caused the patient discomfort. Should they be replaced? Give reasons.

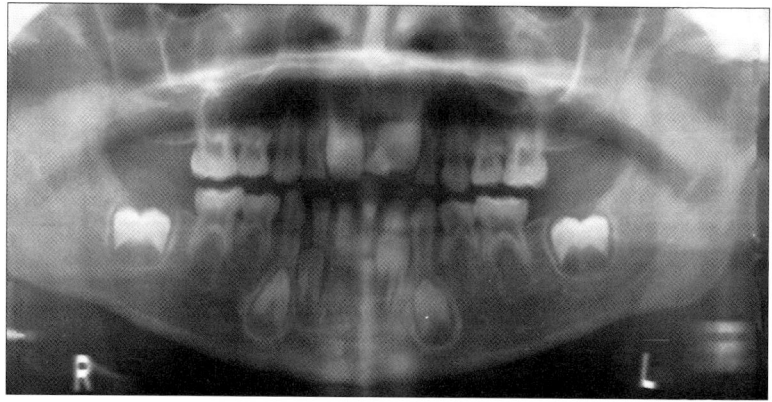

48 (a) What condition can be diagnosed from this dental panoramic tomograph of a 6-year-old patient?
(b) With what condition may it be associated and what are the clinical features?

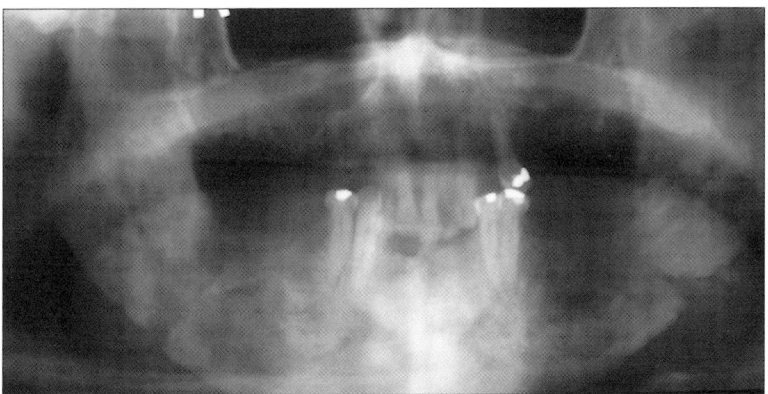

49 This dental panoramic tomograph is of a 65-year-old who had received a course of radiotherapy for a floor-of-mouth carcinoma some 20 years previously. Several posterior teeth had been extracted from both sides of the mandible 3 months before this radiograph was taken.
(a) Describe the radiographic changes in the mandible.
(b) What is the most likely diagnosis?
(c) What other conditions can produce a similar appearance radiographically?

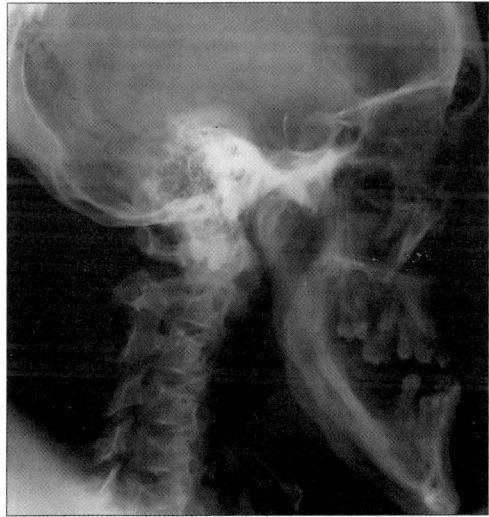

50 A 30-year-old man complained of an alteration in his facial appearance and the way his teeth occluded.
(a) Describe the main abnormalities shown in this lateral skull radiograph.
(b) What is the diagnosis?
(c) What is the cause of the condition?

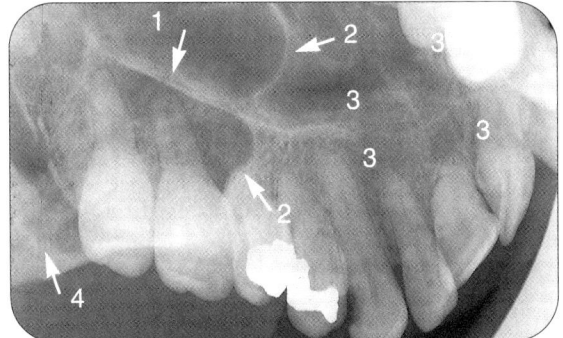

51 What are the anatomical structures identified by **1–4** in this upper oblique occlusal radiograph?

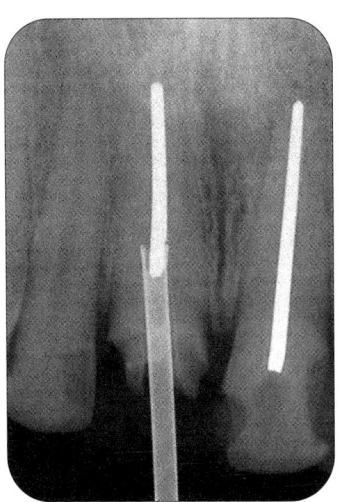

52 (a) What procedure is depicted in this periapical radiograph?
(b) What problems may you anticipate from the radiographic appearance?

53 You are the Radiation Protection Supervisor in a general dental practice. You have been requested to introduce measures to improve radiographic quality. The practice has three dentists, Mr A, Ms B and yourself, each with their own dental X-ray set, and a single darkroom using manual processing. No extra-oral radiographs are taken. Radiography is carried out using the bisecting-angle technique for periapicals. As part of an initial audit of quality, you identify two main problems:
(a) The images in Mr. A's upper molar periapicals are always elongated, with the apices of the teeth frequently missed off.
(b) Ms B complains that sometimes radiographs come out 'completely black'. Describe what could have caused each of these problems and how you would investigate and solve them.

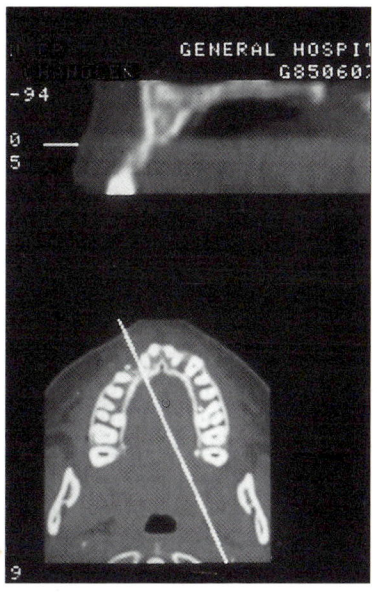

54 The lower part of the illustration shows a slice from a computerized tomographic scan taken in an axial (horizontal) plane through the maxillary canine region at the level of the alveolus. This was taken during the initial assessment phase for placement of a Brånemark osseointegrated implant. The images show that there is sufficient room to place an implant 10 mm in length and of 4 mm diameter. There are no clinical contraindications to the insertion of an implant.
(a) How has the image in the upper part of the illustration been formed?
(b) Assuming you know the crest diameter from the computerized tomographic scans, what further radiographic information is required?

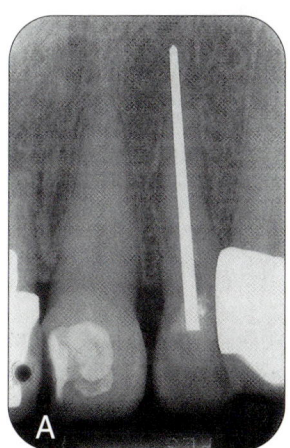

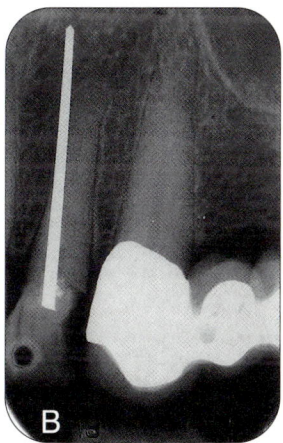

55 Comment on the appearance of the root filling|2̲ .

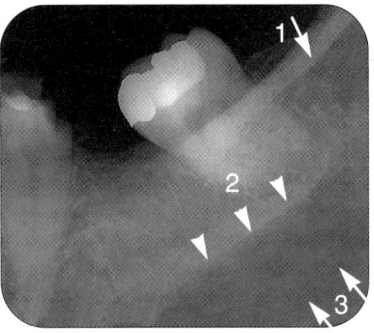

56 (a) What are the anatomical structures 1–3 in this periapical radiograph?
(b) Why is the bone below structure 2 in the right-hand corner of the illustration more radiolucent than bone in most other parts of the film?

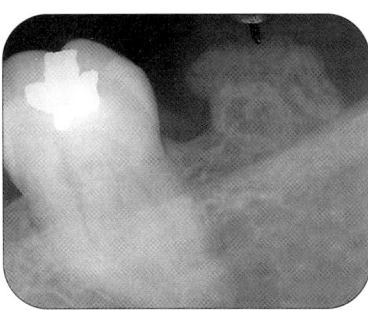

57 What is the differential diagnosis of the exophytic radiopaque mass distal to the lower second molar in this periapical radiograph?

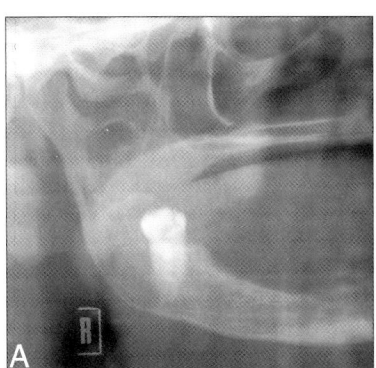

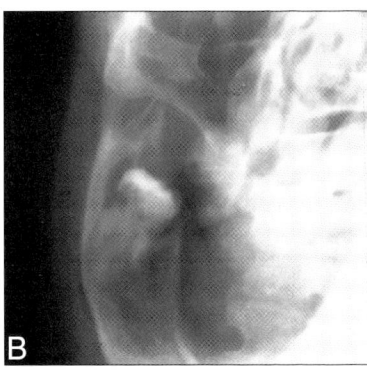

58 This 65-year-old patient complained of recurrent discomfort and discharge in the region of the lower right third molar, beneath a full denture. Initially, a dental panoramic tomograph (58A) was requested.
(a) What are the main radiographic features present?
(b) What type of radiograph is 58B and why was it taken?
(c) What is the differential diagnosis?
(d) Would follow-up radiographs be essential in this patient and, if so, why?

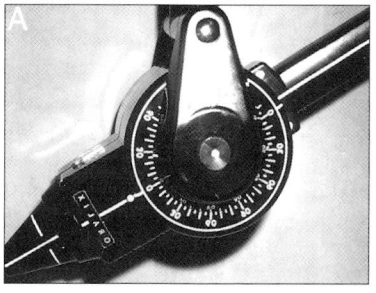
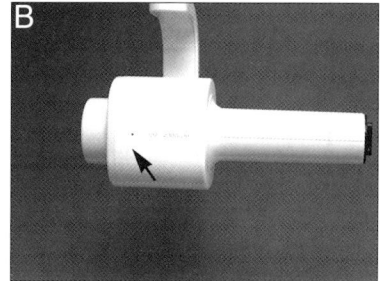

59 What are the differences between the spacer cones on the X-ray sets shown?

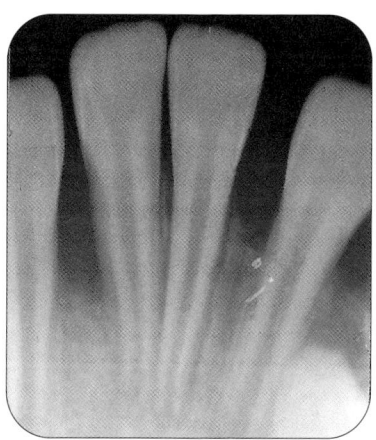

60 This 7 year-old child, with recently erupted lower incisors, complained of slight bleeding from the gums. His general medical history was unremarkable.
(a) What does this periapical radiograph show?
(b) Give a differential diagnosis.

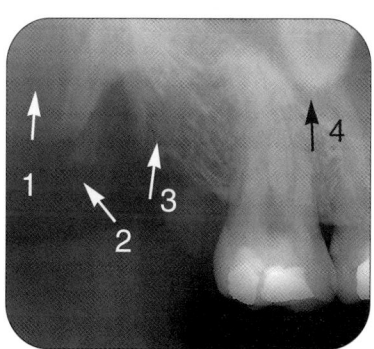

61 What are the anatomical structures identified by **1–4** in this periapical radiograph?

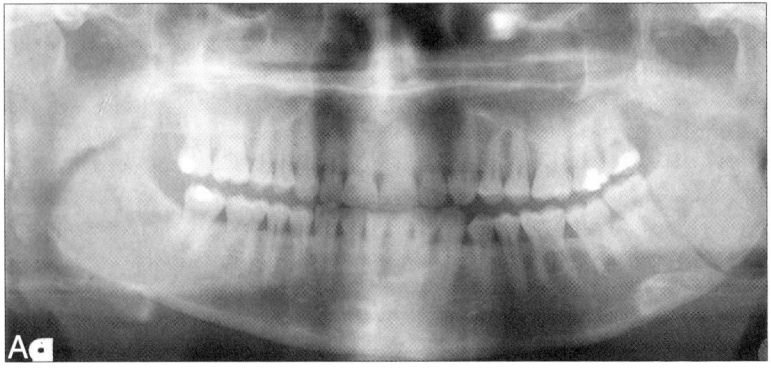

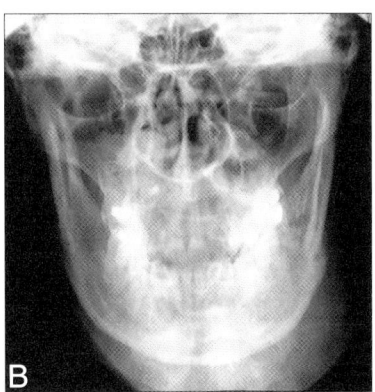

62 (a) Describe the obvious abnormality in the dental panoramic tomograph **62A**.
(b) What additional information may be obtained from the postero-anterior radiograph **62B**?
(c) What other bony injury would you look for on the radiograph?
(d) Outline the management.

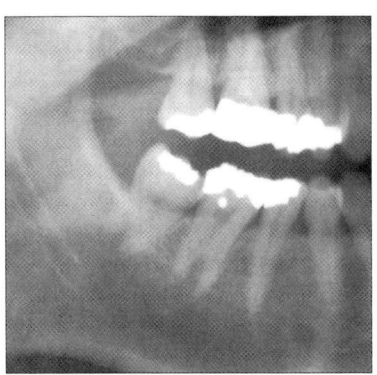

63 (a) Describe the appearance of 6⌐ illustrated in this dental panoramic tomograph.
(b) What abnormality is illustrated?

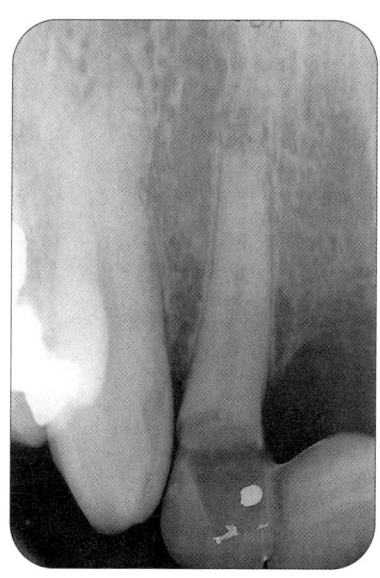

64 This patient complained that his three-unit fixed–fixed ceramic bridge, replacing 1|, was 'loose at one end'. A clinical examination revealed that the porcelain jacket crown retainer at |1 was satisfactory, but there was a gap at the margin of the 2| crown and this part of the bridge could be displaced from the root.
(a) Why is the bridge mobile?
(b) Assuming |1 was sufficient to support the pontic replacing 1|, what treatment would you consider?
(c) What are the dense radiopacities on the incisal edge of the crown preparation?

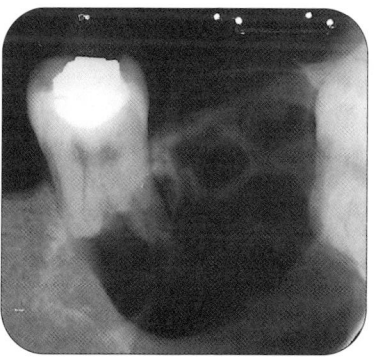

65 This periapical radiograph was taken of a 25-year-old man who complained of a painless swelling of his jaw on the left side.
(a) Describe the lesion shown.
(b) What other radiographic views would be helpful in reaching a diagnosis?
(c) What conditions should be included in the differential diagnosis?

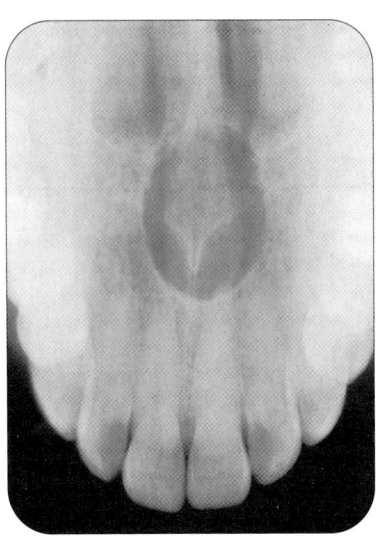

66 This radiograph was taken of a 22-year-old who complained of a nontender palatal swelling, which had been present for several weeks.
(a) What is the radiographic view illustrated?
(b) Describe the abnormality.
(c) What is the 'V'-shaped linear radiopacity lying within the lesion?
(d) What is the most likely diagnosis?
(e) What is the management?

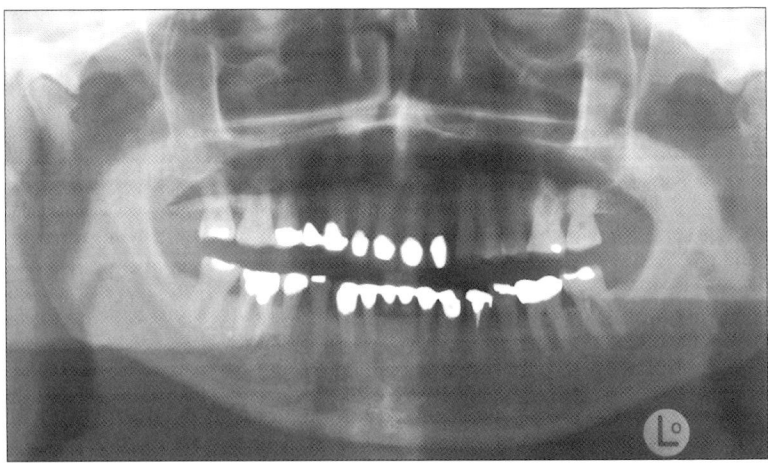

67 This 47-year-old complained of intermittent discomfort affecting the right side of his face. From the evidence presented in the dental panoramic tomograph, what are the possible causes of the symptoms?

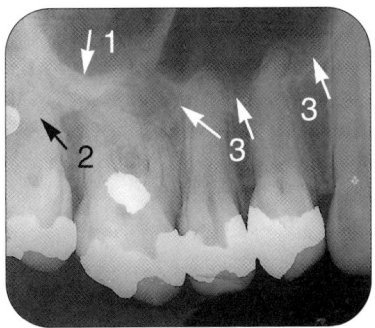

68 What are the anatomical structures identified by 1–3 in this periapical radiograph?

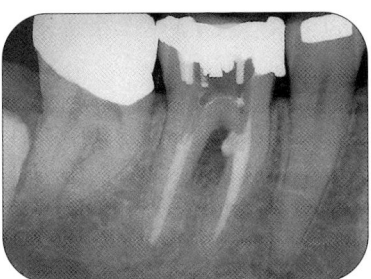

69 (a) What procedural error has occurred in the mesial root of the lower right first molar, as shown on this periapical radiograph?
(b) How may this be managed?

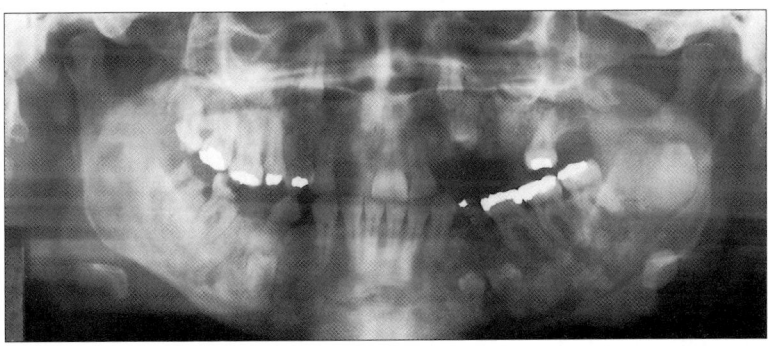

70 This 30-year-old patient requested treatment of her painful decayed lower right molar teeth.
(a) Describe the radiological abnormalities in this dental panoramic tomograph.
(b) What is the most probable cause of her discomfort?
(c) What is the most likely diagnosis of the condition illustrated?
(d) What further investigations should be performed?

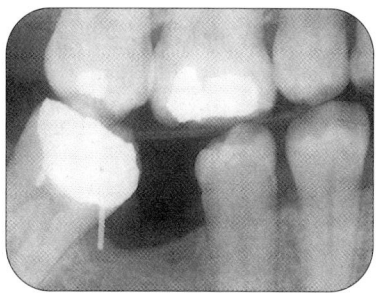 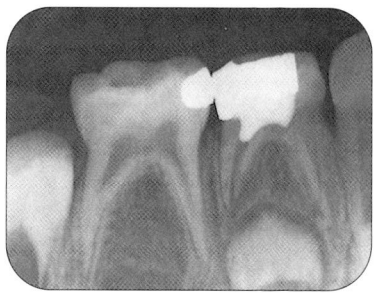

71 (a) What abnormality of $\overline{7|}$ is shown on this bitewing radiograph?
(b) Why is this most likely to have occurred?
(c) How might the abnormality have been avoided?
(d) What is the management?

72 (a) What does this periapical radiograph show?
(b) What is the approximate age of this patient?
(c) Is the second premolar absent?

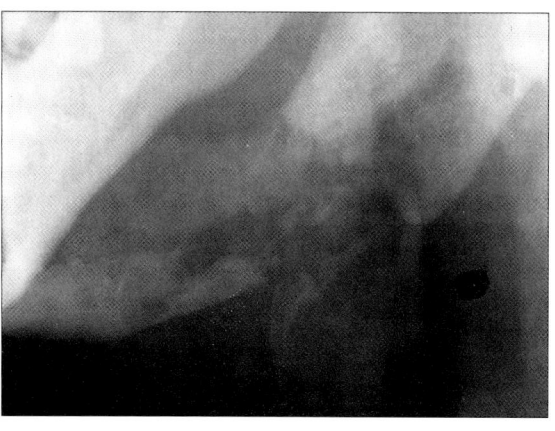

73 This oblique lateral radiograph of the mandible was taken of a 70-year-old diabetic man who complained of severe pain with facial swelling on the left side. He had attended a dentist 6 weeks previously for the removal of a infected left lower molar tooth.
(a) Describe the radiographic appearance of the mandible.
(b) What is the most likely diagnosis?
(c) What other lesions can produce a similar radiographic appearance?
(d) What is the radiopaque structure marked by arrow?

74 Under what conditions would you use a lead protective apron for a patient undergoing intra-oral dental radiography?

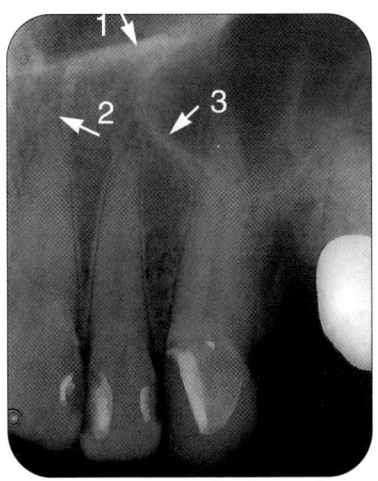

75 Identify the structures labelled **1–3** in this periapical radiograph.

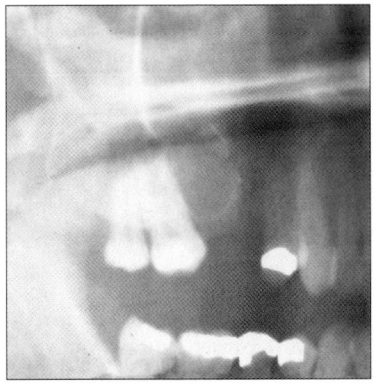

76 This dental panoramic tomograph was taken 3 weeks after the extraction of the root-filled 5|, because of persistent postoperative discomfort and failure of the socket to heal.
(a) What abnormality is present that may account for the symptoms?
(b) What further radiographs may be helpful and why?
(c) What is the management?

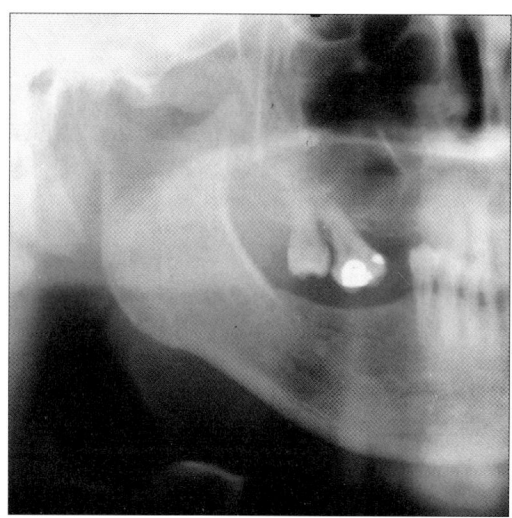

77 A 40-year-old woman heard a crack in her right ear during mastication. She then developed pain in the preauricular region and limitation in opening her mouth.
(a) What abnormalities are present in the dental panoramic tomograph?
(b) What is the most likely diagnosis?
(c) What further investigations are indicated and why?

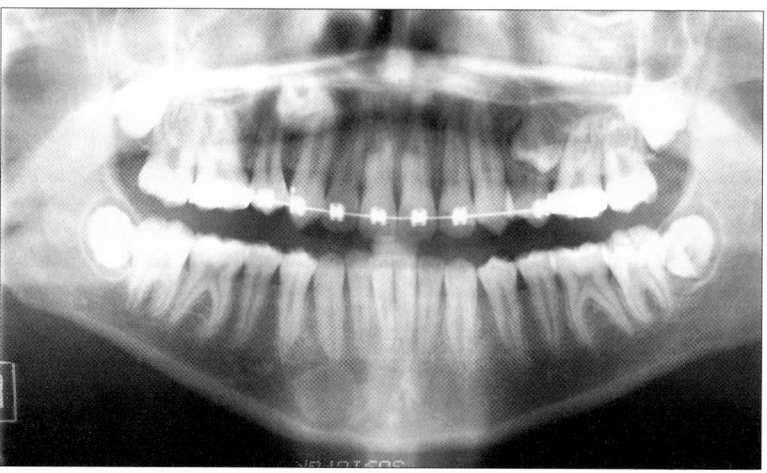

78 (a) What is the approximate age of this patient and what treatment is being undertaken?
(b) Describe the unerupted teeth.
(c) How may the unerupted teeth affect the outcome of the treatment?
(d) Describe the appearance of the bone in the lower right canine region and what is the diagnosis?

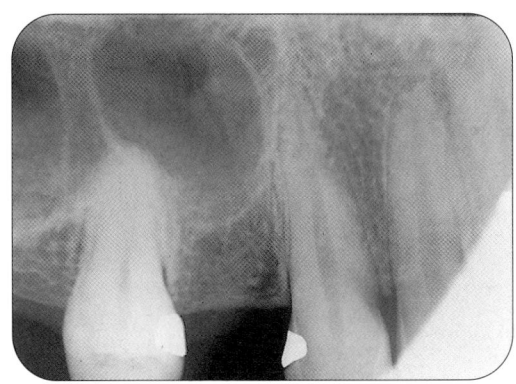

79 (a) What is the cause of the radiolucency between the apices of 5| and 3| in this periapical radiograph?
(b) What radiographic technical errors are present?

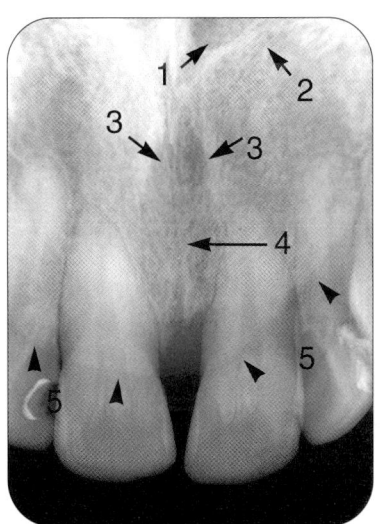

80 What are the anatomical structures identified by **1–5** in this periapical radiograph?

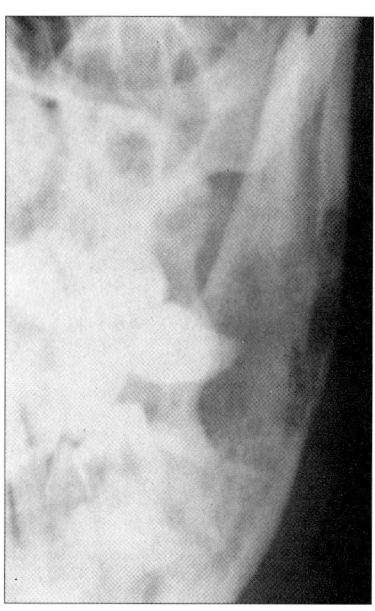

81 This postero-anterior radiograph of the mandible was taken of a 57-year-old woman who complained of a reduction of sensation in her lower lip on the left side.
(a) Describe the abnormal radiographic appearance illustrated.
(b) What is the most likely diagnosis?
(c) What further images of the jaw lesion would be helpful?
(d) What subsequent investigation would help determine whether other bone lesions are present?
(e) What other conditions can produce a similar radiographic appearance?

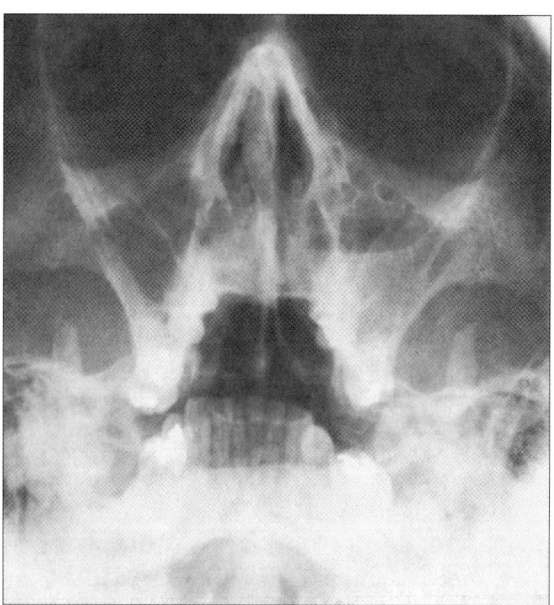

82 This patient, who had the 6 extracted 2 weeks before, complains of a throbbing left-sided facial pain and failure of the tooth socket to heal.
(a) What abnormality is shown on this occipitomental radiograph?
(b) What is its probable cause?
(c) What is the management?

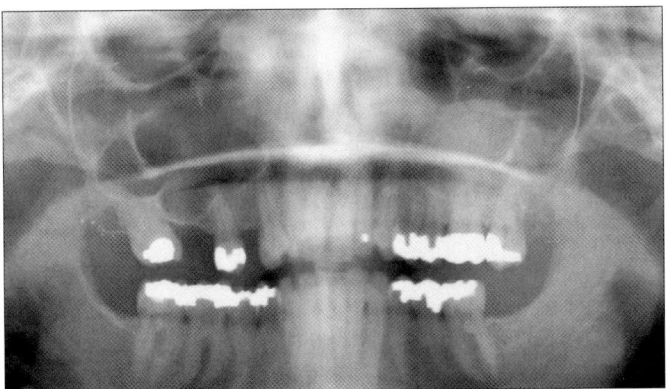

83 This dental panoramic tomograph was taken of a 29-year-old patient.
(a) Describe the abnormality affecting the left maxillary antrum.
(b) What is the most likely diagnosis?
(c) What is the differential diagnosis?
(d) What is the management?

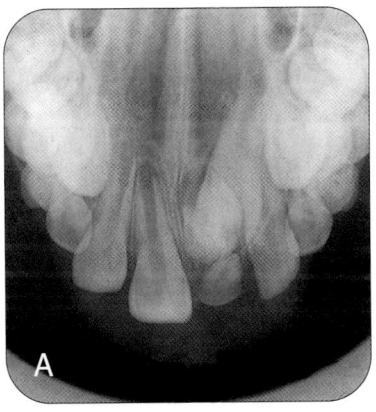 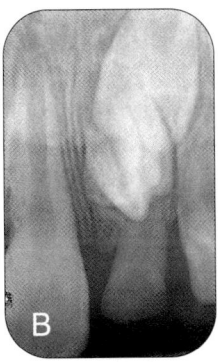

84 The mother of this 8-year-old boy was concerned that his upper left permanent central incisor had not erupted and that the primary incisor was still present.
(a) Which radiographic views are shown ?
(b) What is the reason for the delayed eruption of the central incisor?
(c) What treatment is required?

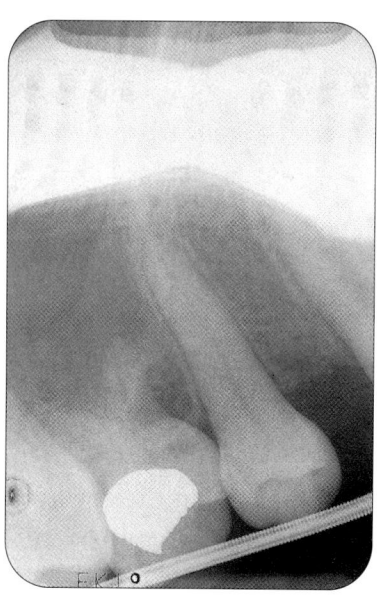

85 This periapical radiograph of E4| was taken using the bisecting angle technique.
(a) What faults are shown?
(b) How might they have been avoided?

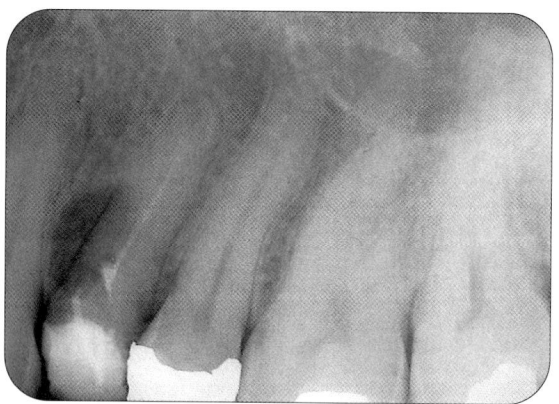

86 The patient (aged 32 years) complained of a recurrent buccal swelling associated with the left upper first premolar.
(a) Describe the abnormalities associated with this tooth on this periapical radiograph.
(b) How may the condition be managed?

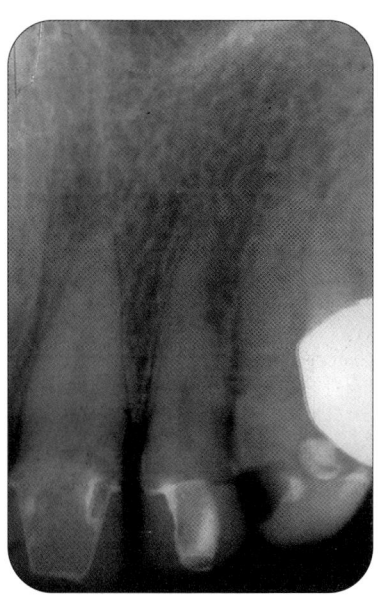

87 This patient has porcelain jacket crowns⎢12, and endodontic treatment is required for⎢2 because it is associated with a buccally discharging sinus.
(a) What complicating factors might you encounter?
(b) What steps would you take to overcome them?

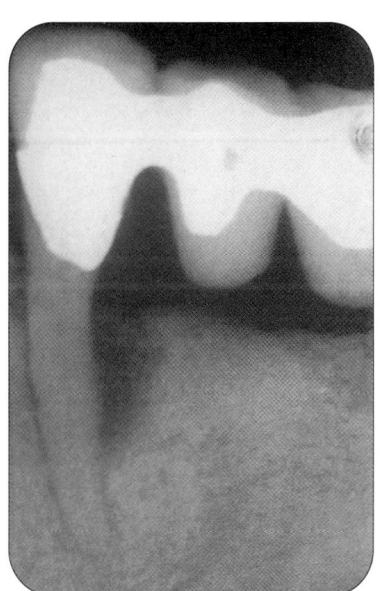

88 This 45-year-old patient has a severe vertical bone defect, which was found to be three-walled, distally to his lower left first premolar.
(a) Can this deduction be made from the periapical radiograph shown?
(b) What is the most likely cause of the defect?
(c) What would be the most suitable treatment?

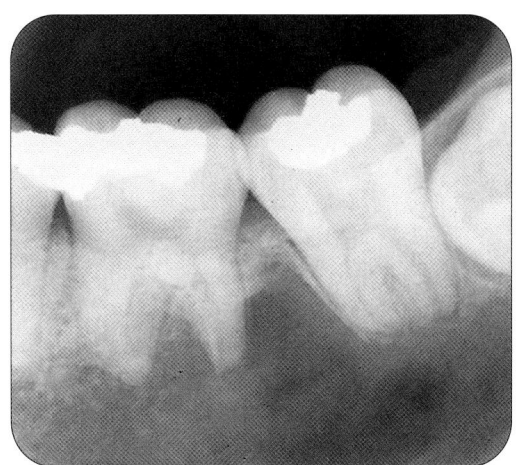

89 The radiolucency on this periapical radiograph of the lower left molar region was discovered as an incidental finding in a 16-year-old girl.
(a) What other radiographic views would you take?
(b) Describe the radiographic appearance of the lesion.
(c) What is the most likely diagnosis?

Added filtration	Main beam dose rate (mGys–1)	Skin dose (mGy)	Exposure time (s)
Nil	17.9	8.2	0.45
1.1 mm Al	6.1	3.5	0.55

90 Explain the significance of the data in the table above.
Al, Aluminium.

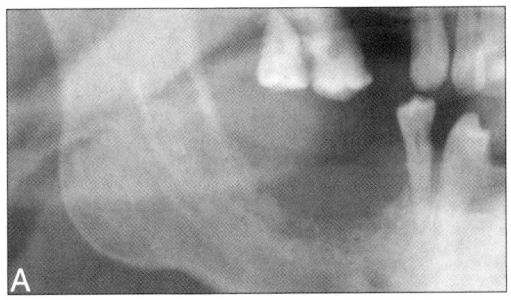

91 A 64-year-old male, who was a heavy drinker and smoker, complained of a painful ulcer in the right side of the floor of his mouth and right alveolus. The dental panoramic tomograph **91A** shows a poorly defined area of bone destruction in the right molar region of the mandible. Further investigations were undertaken.

(a) What type of investigation is illustrated in **91B**?

(b) What abnormality is visible?

(c) What type of investigation is shown in **91C**?

(d) What abnormality is visible?

(e) What is the most likely diagnosis?

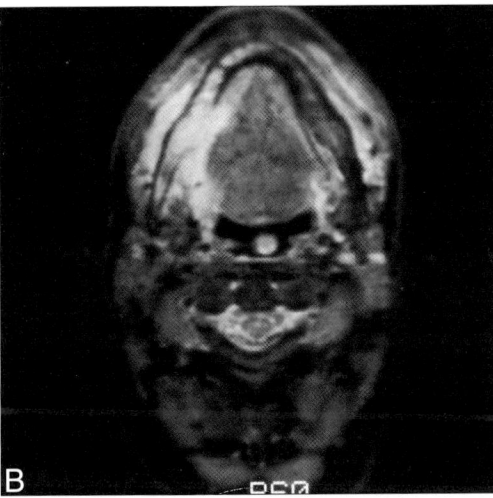

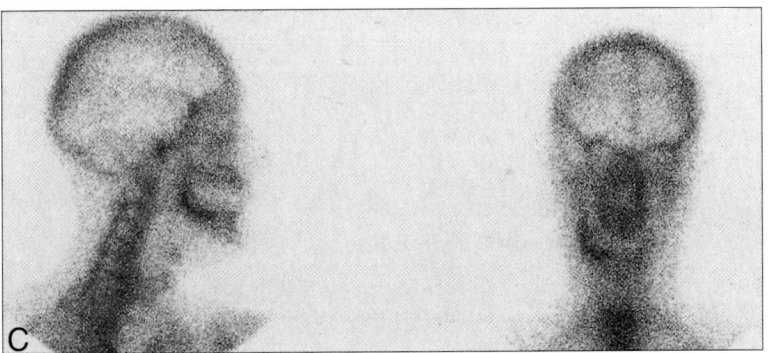

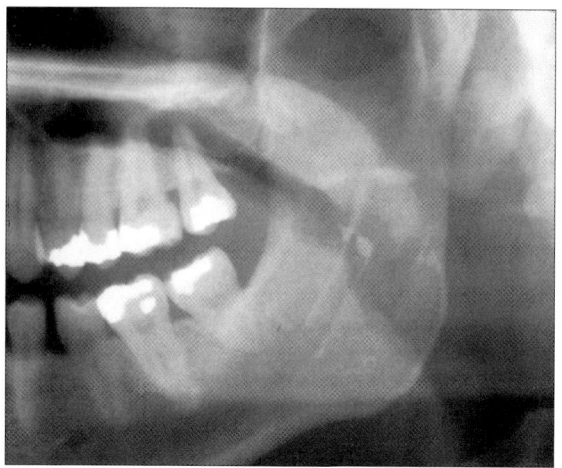

92 What are the three abnormal radiopacities illustrated on this dental panoramic tomograph?

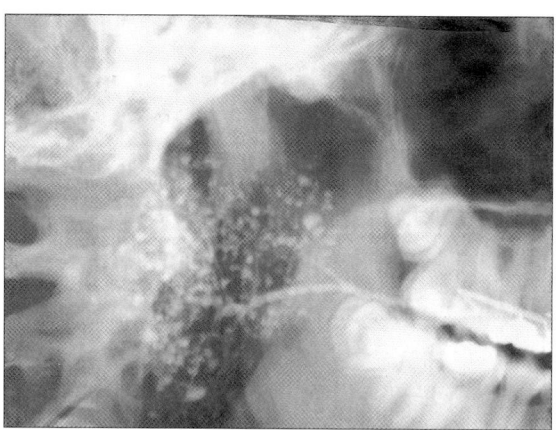

93 (a) What type of radiographic investigation is shown?
(b) What are the main indications for this investigation?
(c) What abnormality is shown?

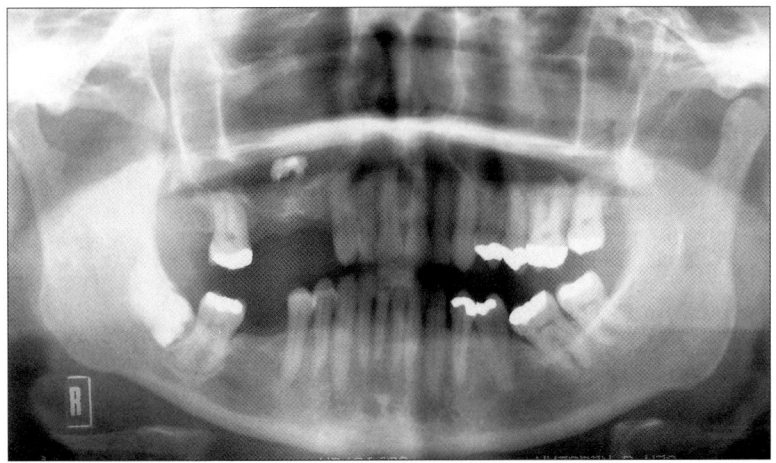

94 This routine dental panoramic tomograph contains a chance finding in the upper right quadrant.
(a) Describe the abnormality.
(b) What is the diagnosis and how may the clinical history assist a diagnosis?
(c) What further radiographic views are required and why?

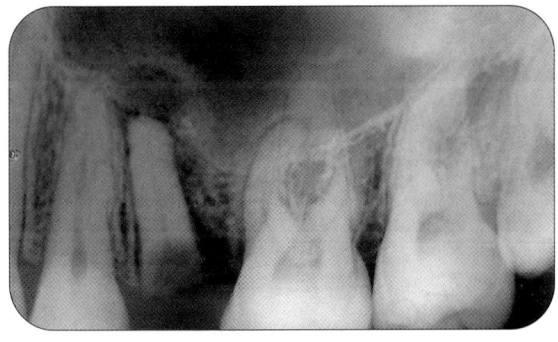

95 This patient requested a bridge to replace 5
Examination revealed the presence of a retained root.
(a) Describe the changes associated with the root on this periapical radiograph.
(b) What is the differential diagnosis of the condition?
(c) What particular complications may arise if the root is removed?

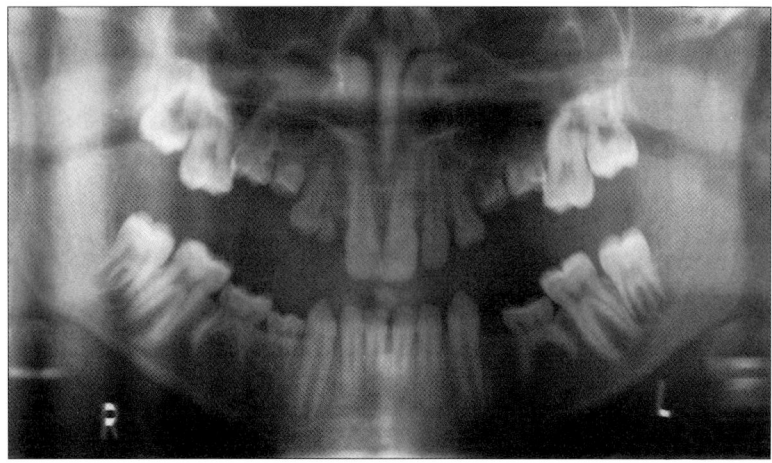

96 This 13-year-old patient was referred for advice concerning the delay in eruption of his permanent teeth.
(a) What are the main abnormalities shown in this dental panoramic tomograph?
(b) What is the prognosis for his teeth?
(c) Outline the management.

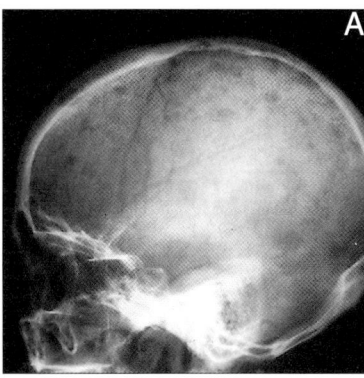

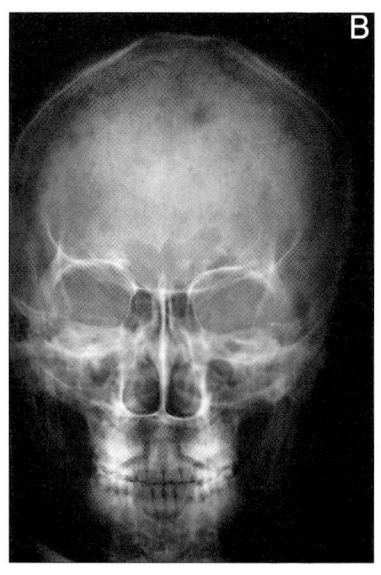

97 (a) What two radiographic views are illustrated?
(b) What abnormalities do they show?
(c) What is the most likely diagnosis?

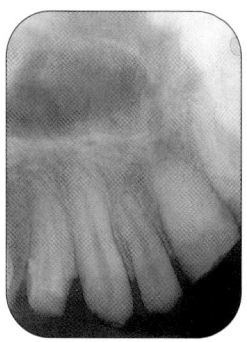 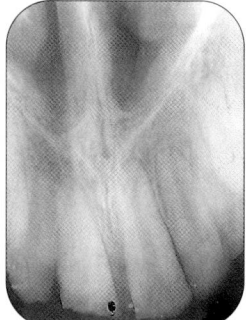 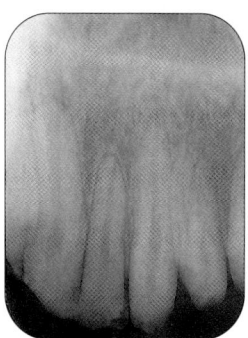

98 This teenager was concerned about the appearance of his teeth.
(a) Describe the abnormalities in these periapical radiographs.
(b) What is the diagnosis?
(c) What is the most likely explanation for the changes in 1⏌?

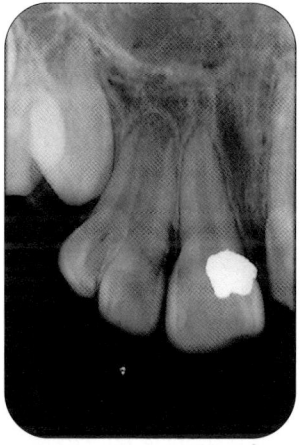

99 (a) Describe the main abnormality in this periapical radiograph.
(b) What is the diagnosis?

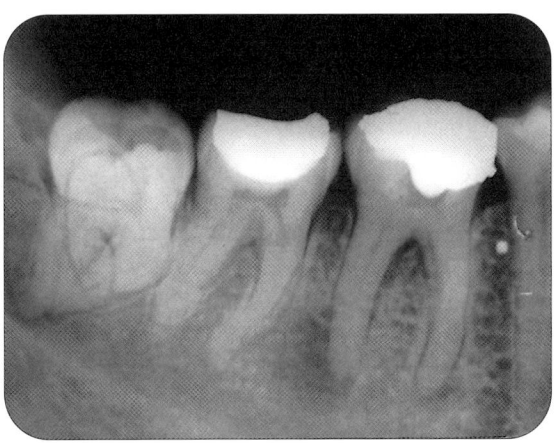

100 This patient complained of persistent severe toothache. The $\overline{6}$ was tender to percussion and clinical examination revealed that the tooth was nonvital.
(a) What is the most likely diagnosis?
(b) Describe the main radiographic appearance associated with $\overline{6}$.
(c) What is the differential diagnosis of the periapical lesions?

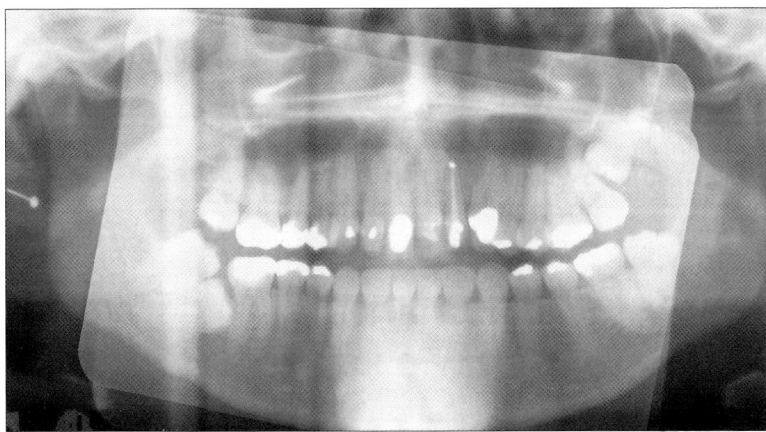

101 What faults are present on this dental panoramic tomograph and how did they arise?

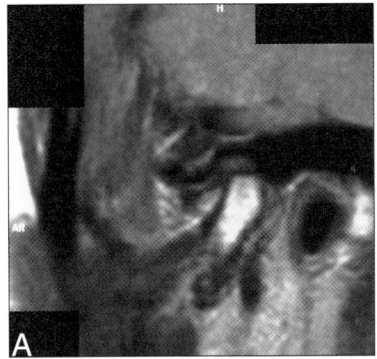
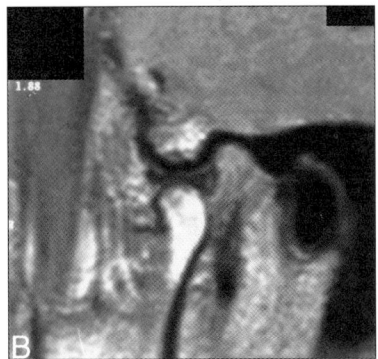

102 This patient suffered with discomfort of several months duration from the right TMJ. It was tender on palpation and a 'click' could be felt on opening. In 102A the mouth is in the closed position and in **102B** it is fully open
(a) What type of imaging technique is shown?
(b) Describe the main abnormality.
(c) What is the condition?

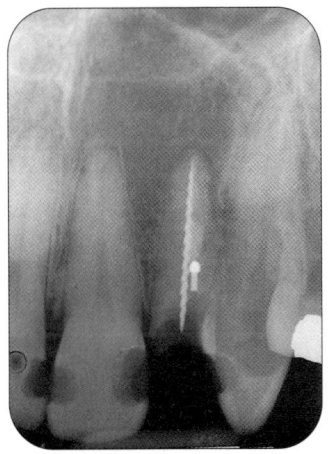

103 (a) Describe the abnormalities on this periapical radiograph.
(b) What is the probable diagnosis?
(c) What clinical sequence of events may have led to the radiographic appearance of the upper left lateral incisor?

104 What, in the United Kingdom, is the difference between a Radiation Protection Supervisor (RPS) and a Radiation Protection Advisor (RPA) regarding qualifications, statutory requirements and duties in the context of general dental practice?

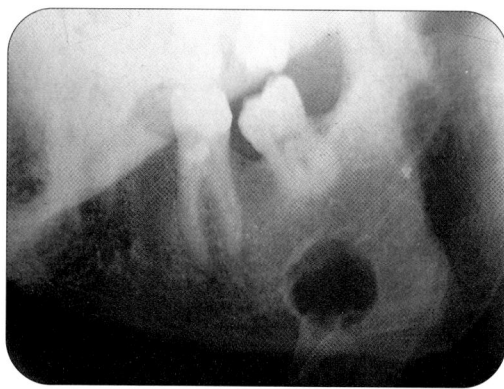

105 The radiolucent lesion on this oblique lateral radiograph of the mandible was discovered as an incidental finding.
(a) Describe the radiographic features of the lesion.
(b) What is the most likely diagnosis?
(c) What further investigation may be useful?

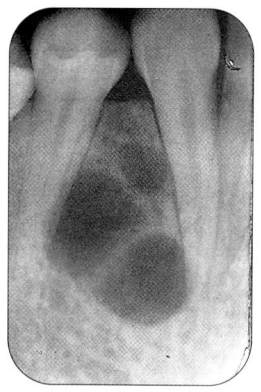

106 This patient has slight buccal expansion of the right side of the mandible.
(a) Describe the lesion in this periapical radiograph.
(b) What is the differential diagnosis?
(c) How would you investigate the condition further?

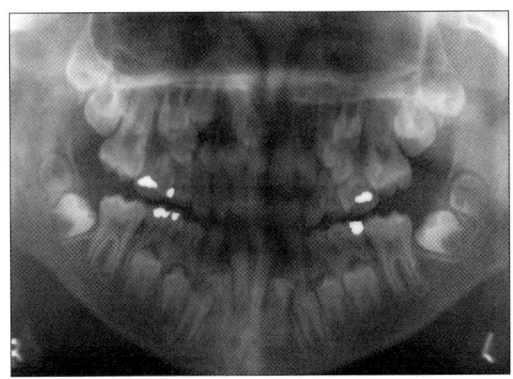

107 This dental panoramic tomograph was taken of a 12-year-old patient.
(a) What abnormalities does it show?
(b) What is the most likely diagnosis and what are the features of this condition?
(c) What is the management?

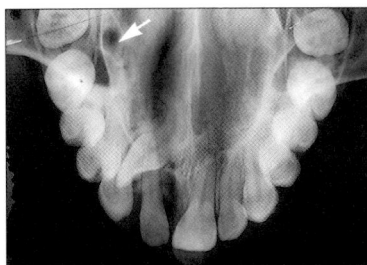

108 (a) What condition is shown in this upper anterior occlusal radiograph?
(b) How might it have arisen?
(c) What is the management?
(d) What is the circular radioucency indicated by the arrow?

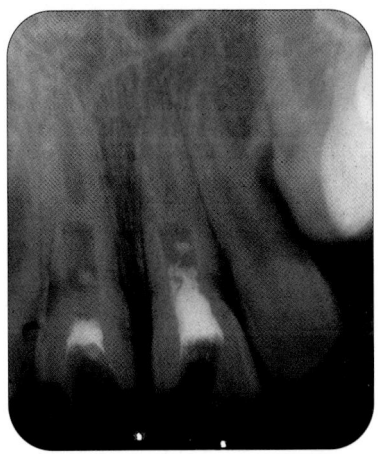

109 This patient requests restoration of 1|1 , which are discoloured and contain defective composite restorations.
(a) Describe the appearance of 1|1 on this periapical radiograph.
(b) Why is there a calcific barrier at midroot level in both teeth?
(c) Outline how this situation might be managed.

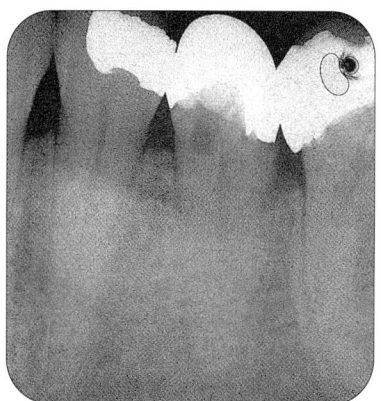

110 (a) Describe the radiopacity overlying on $\overline{45}$ this periapical radiograph?
(b) What is its most likely cause?
(c) What is the differential diagnosis?

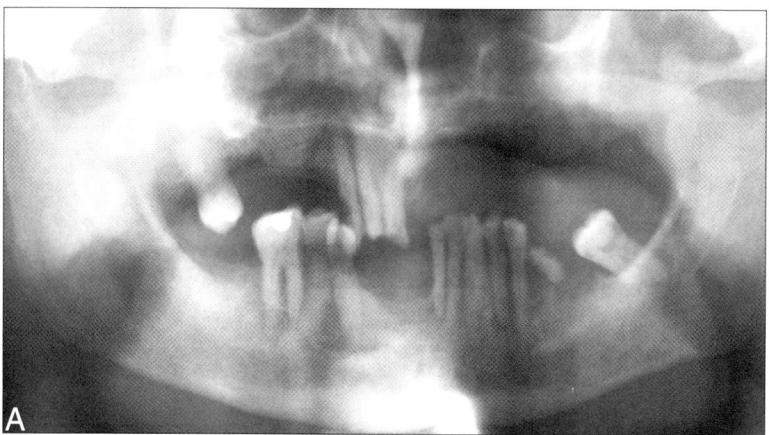

A

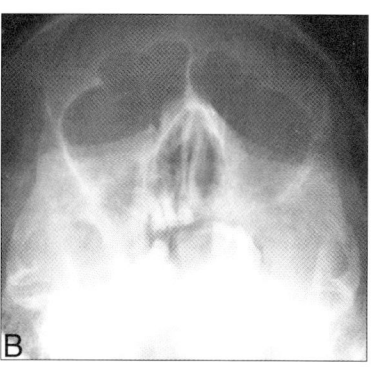

B

111 This elderly patient with neglected teeth complained of pain and swelling in the mouth and around the left cheek.
(a) Describe the radiographic abnormalities affecting the upper left maxilla.
(b) What is the most likely diagnosis and what additional clinical features may be present in this condition?
(c) What further investigations are indicated?

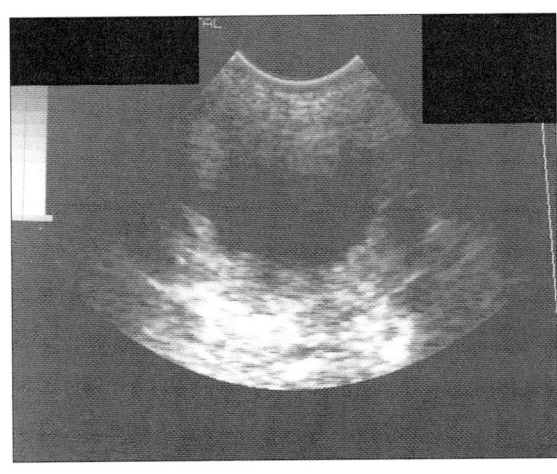

112 This patient complained of a large smooth swelling in the floor of the mouth, and some difficulty with swallowing.
(a) What investigation is illustrated?
(b) How is the image formed?
(c) What type of condition is shown?

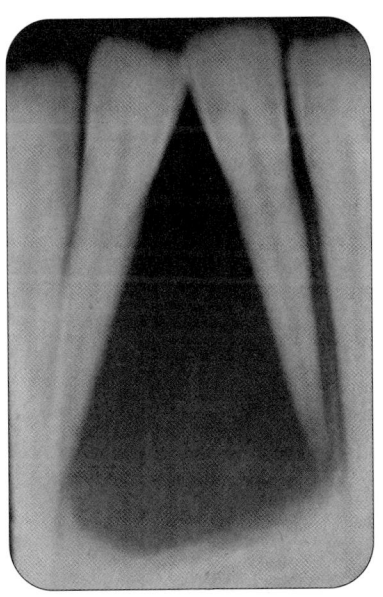

113 This is a periapical radiograph of the lower incisors of a 14-year-old who complained of a slowly enlarging lump in the midline of the mandible. The lower incisor teeth were vital.
(a) Describe the radiographic features of this lesion.
(b) What conditions should be included in a differential diagnosis?
(c) What other investigations would you request and why?

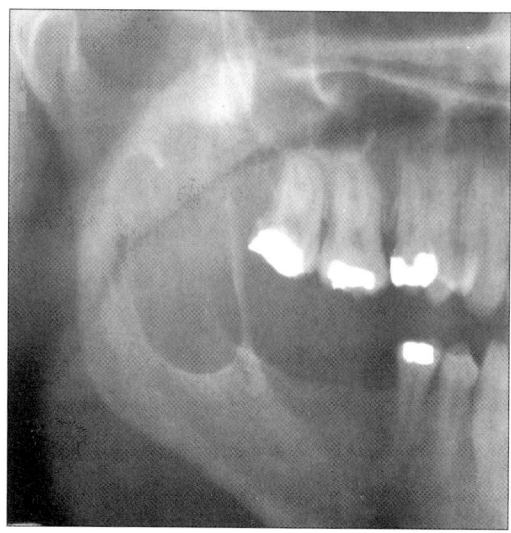

114 This 39-year-old patient complained of acute discomfort and swelling of sudden onset affecting the cheek and mandible on the right side.
(a) Describe the abnormality shown on the dental panoramic tomograph.
(b) What is the most likely diagnosis of this abnormality?

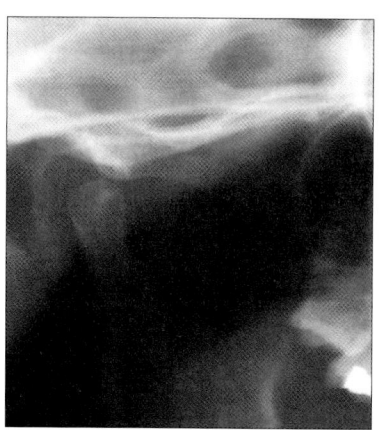 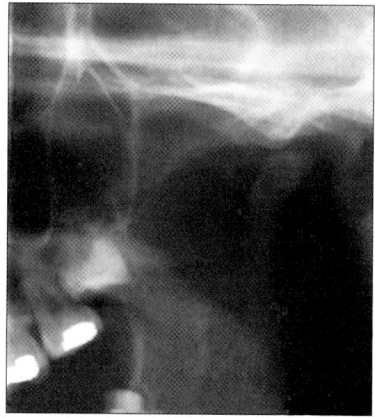

115 (a) What type of radiographs are illustrated?
(b) What abnormalities are visible?
(c) What is the most likely diagnosis?
(d) What are the most common clinical features associated with this condition?
(e) What other radiographic features can be found in this disorder?

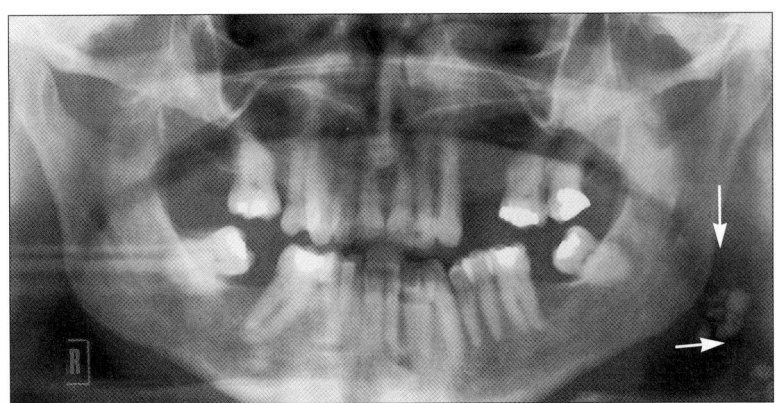

116 (a) Describe the radiopacities arrowed in this dental panoramic tomograph.
(b) What is the most likely diagnosis?
(c) What are the horizontal linear radiopaque lines on the opposite side of the radiograph?

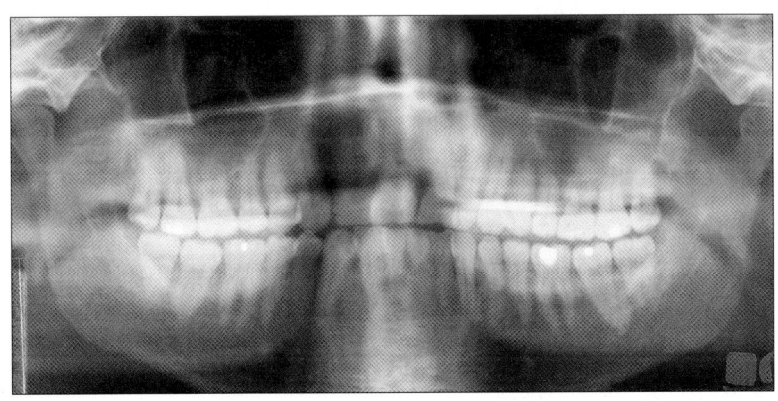

117 (a) What error is present on this dental panoramic tomograph?
(b) Describe how the fault can be avoided.

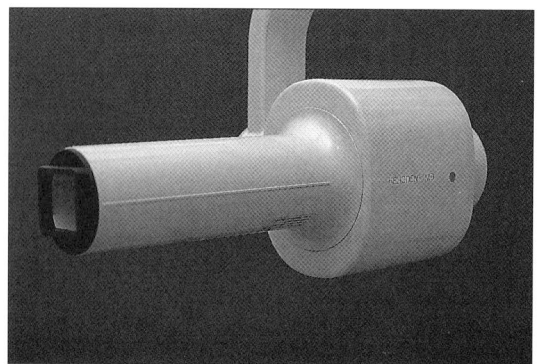

118 Comment on the appearence of the cone-end on this dental X-ray set.

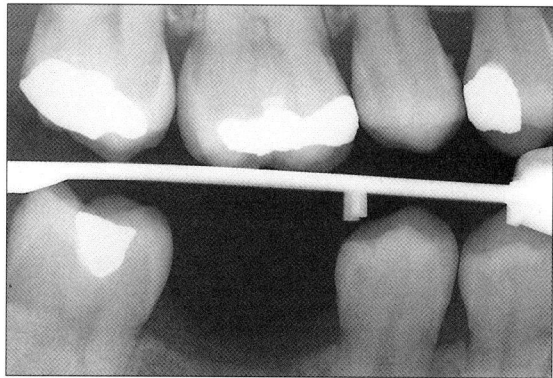

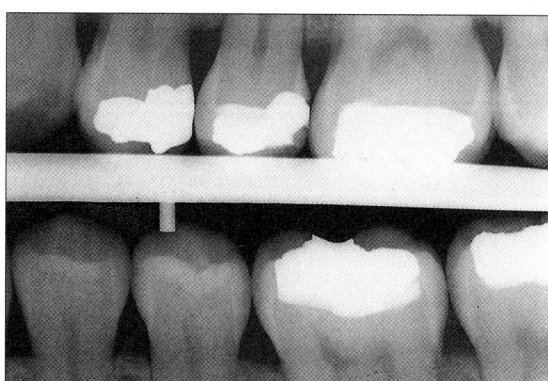

119 (a) What technique has been used in the restorations that have been placed in the distal aspects of the upper right and left second premolar teeth, shown on these bitewing radiographs? (b) What factors account for the different radiographic appearances in the two teeth?

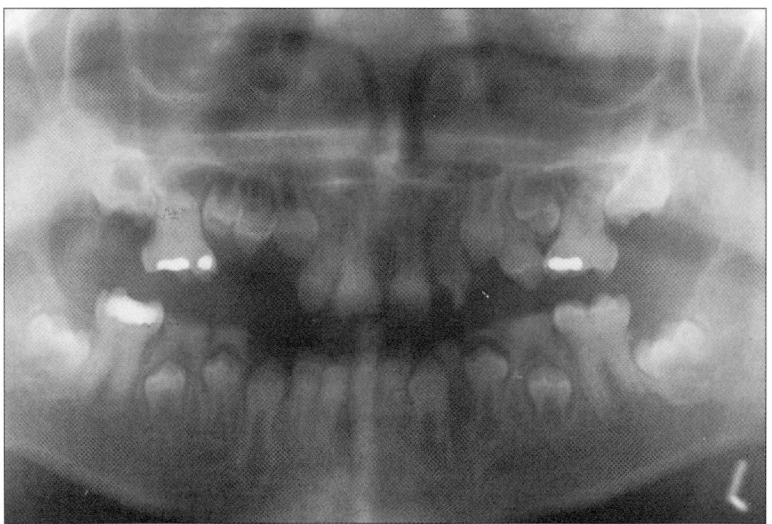

120 (a) What would be this boy's most likely complaint and why?
(b) What abnormalities of the dentition are apparent on this dental panoramic tomograph?
(c) What would be the histological appearance of the teeth?

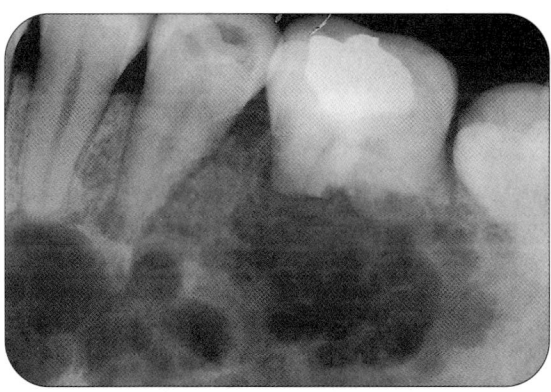

121 This periapical radiograph was taken of a 32-year-old Nigerian who had a slowly enlarging swelling of the left side of the jaw.
(a) Describe the radiographic appearance of the lesion.
(b) What is the differential diagnosis.

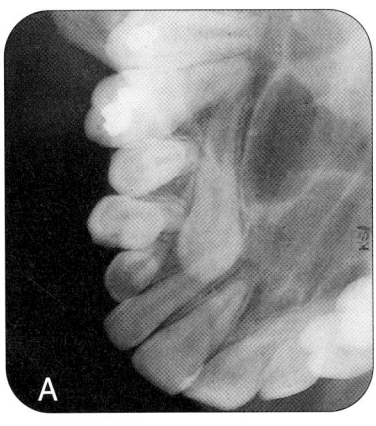

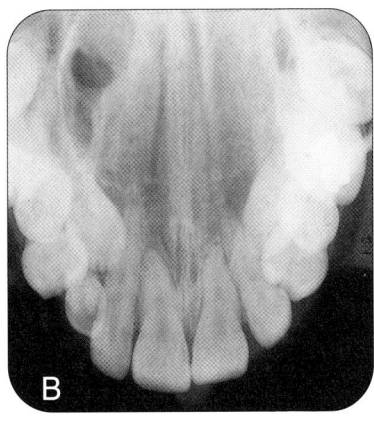

122 A clinical examination of this patient revealed that <u>3</u>|had not erupted.
(a) What radiographic views are illustrated?
(b) Does the unerupted <u>3</u>| lie buccally or palatally in the dental arch? Explain.

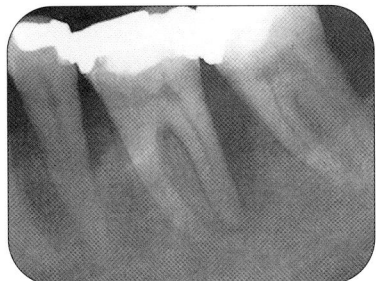

123 This periapical radiograph is of a 46-year-old woman.
(a) Describe the abnormalities.
(b) What is the diagnosis?
(c) What are the treatment options available for the first molar?

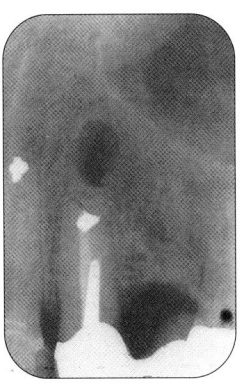

124 This periapical radiograph was taken 2 years after apical surgery and cyst enucleation |1 2 .
(a) Outline the radiographic features of |2
(b) What is the most likely diagnosis of the radiolucency|2 ?
(c) What is the management?

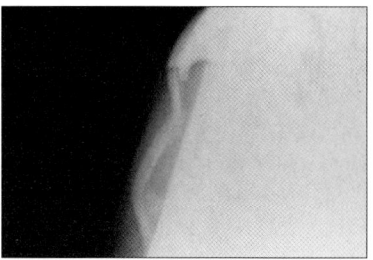

125 This patient suffered a blow to the right side of his face.
(a) What is the radiographic view illustrated?
(b) What abnormality is present?
(c) What are the cardinal signs and symptoms of this condition?
(d) Outline the management.

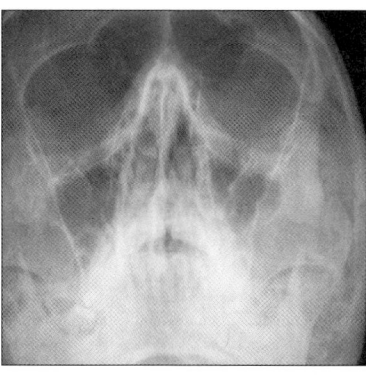

126 This occipitomental radiograph was taken after an assault.
(a) What effects of the trauma are shown?
(b) List the patient's likely symptoms and clinical signs.
(c) What further radiographic or imaging investigations may be undertaken in a patient with this type of injury, and why?

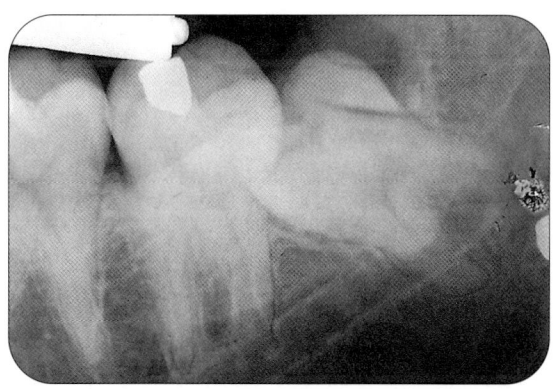

127 This patient seeks your advice regarding episodes of discomfort in the lower left molar region.
(a) What might be the cause of the symptoms?
(b) What is the likely management of this patient?

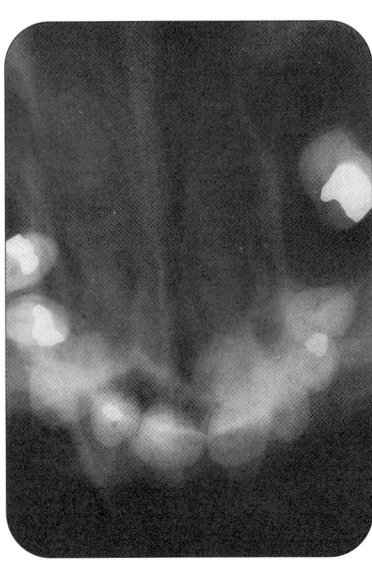

128 This patient is concerned about the appearance of her upper left maxillary canine.
(a) What type of radiographic view is shown?
(b) How is it taken?
(c) What abnormality is shown?
(d) What are the disadvantages of this radiographic technique?

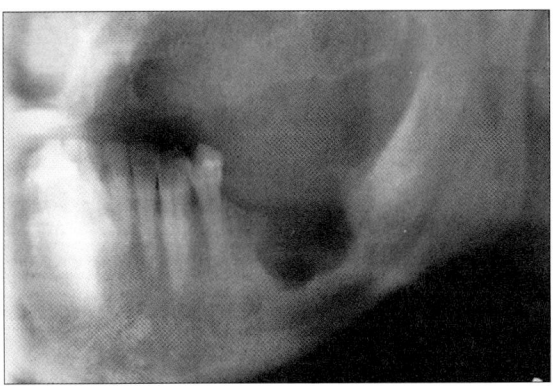

129 This oblique lateral radiograph of the mandible of a 30-year-old patient was taken 2 days after a general dental practitioner had extracted 6 . The caries-free tooth was, apparently, floating or standing in space because of extensive resorption of the surrounding bone.
(a) Describe the radiographic appearance of this lesion.
(b) What is the differential diagnosis?

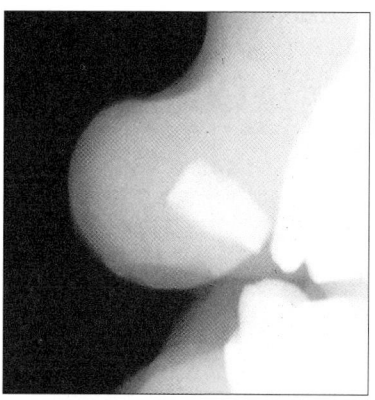

130 This patient was struck in the face by a hockey stick.
(a) What is the radiographic view shown?
(b) What abnormality is illustrated?

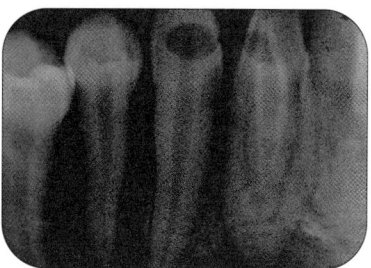

131 This is a periapical radiograph of the $\overline{54321}$ region.
(a) Describe the radiographic features associated with $\overline{2}$.
(b) What is the condition?
(c) What is the radiolucent defect present in the crown $\overline{3}$.

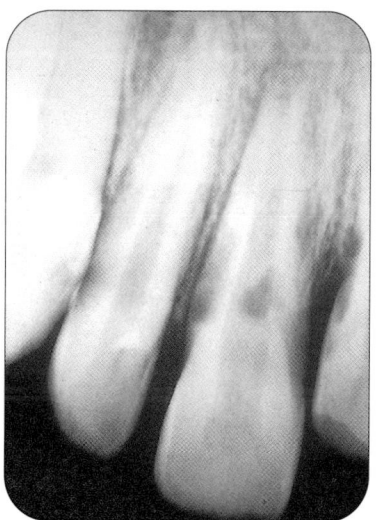

132 This right upper central incisor was avulsed in a bicycle accident 3 years previously and was reimplanted within 2 hours.
(a) What condition is apparent on this periapical radiograph?
(b) What additional treatment should have been carried out?
(c) What factors affect the prognosis for reimplanted teeth?

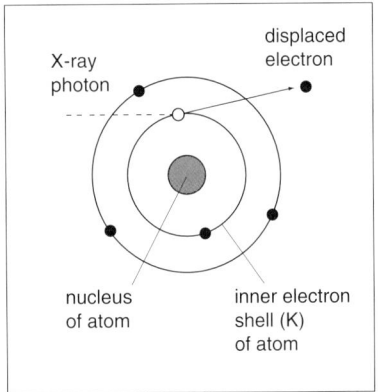

133 (a) What X-ray photon interaction is illustrated here? (b).What factors influence this type of interaction of X-ray photons with matter?

134 This oblique lateral radiograph of the mandible is almost unreadable. (a) Describe the appearance of the radiograph and identify the fault? (b) What are the most likely causes of this appearance? (c) What procedures would you undertake to determine the cause?

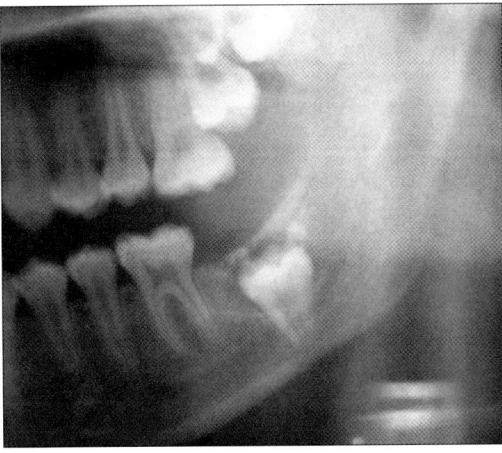

135 The illustration shows part of a dental panoramic radiograph of a 15-year-old. (a) Describe the abnormal radiographic findings. (b) What are the most likely diagnoses?

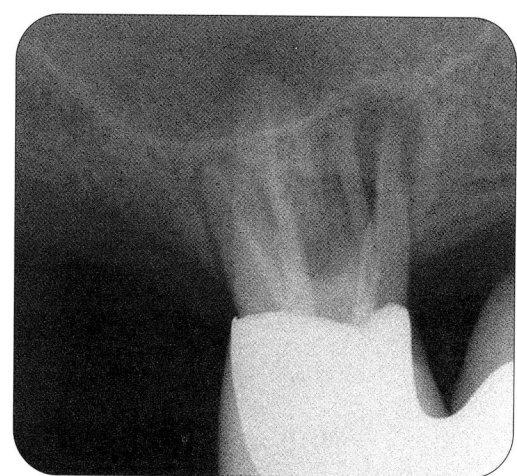

136 (a) Describe the radiographic changes associated with the roots of the upper right molar tooth on this periapical radiograph.
(b) Outline the management.

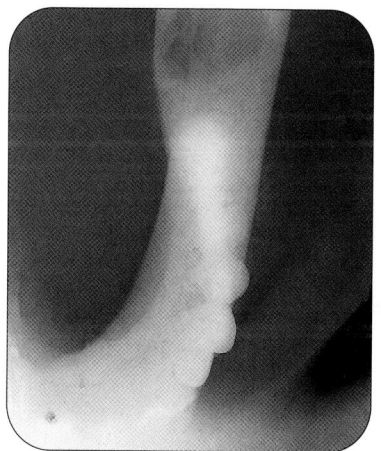

137 This 26-year-old woman presented with pain after extraction of the mandibular second molar.
(a) What is this radiographic view illustrated?
(b) Describe the radiographic feature shown in the first molar and second premolar regions.
(c) What is the differential diagnosis of this appearance?
(d) What other abnormalities can be seen on this radiograph?

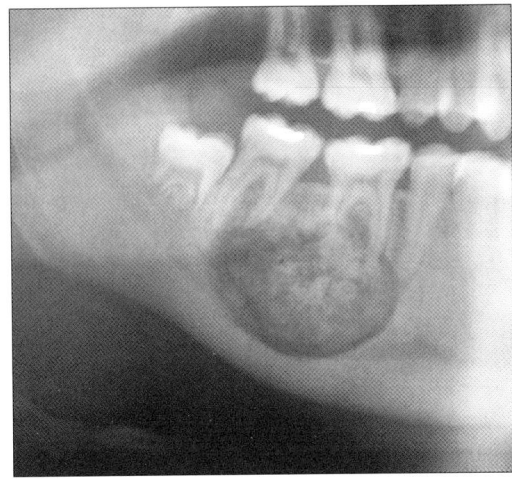

138 This dental panoramic tomograph was taken to investigate a swelling in the $\overline{6|}$ region in a 16-year-old.
(a) Describe the abnormal radiographic appearance.
(b) What is the most likely diagnosis?
(c) What is the management?

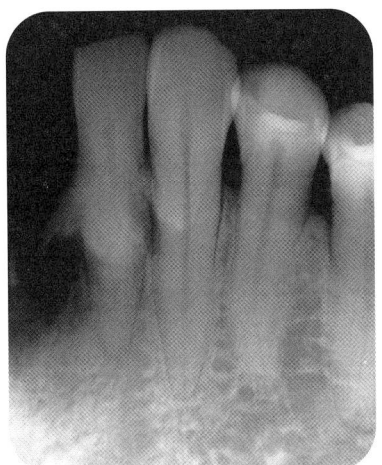
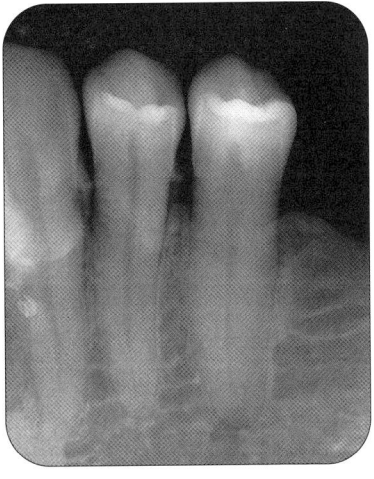

139 (a) What is the cause of the radiopacities overlying the roots of $\overline{|234}$ on these periapical radiographs?
(b) What is the radiolucency at the apex of$\overline{|5}$?

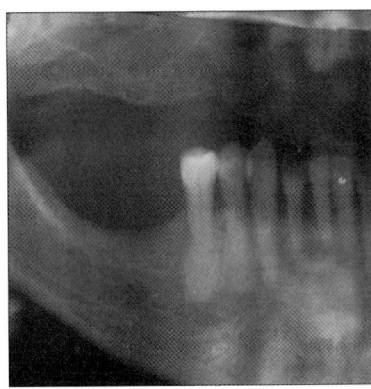

140 (a) What condition affecting
5⌐ is illustrated in this dental
panoramic tomograph?
(b) What are the causes?
(c) What systemic disorders may be
associated with this condition?

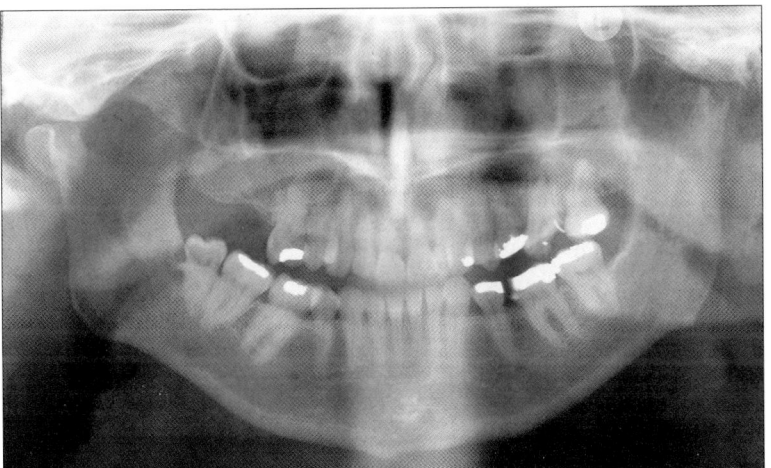

141 This patient fell on the point of his chin, causing a deep laceration of
the skin. A precautionary dental panoramic tomograph was taken.
(a) What features consistent with the history are present?
(b) Might there be any associated dental abnormalities in a patient with this
type of injury?
(c) What further radiographs might be helpful?

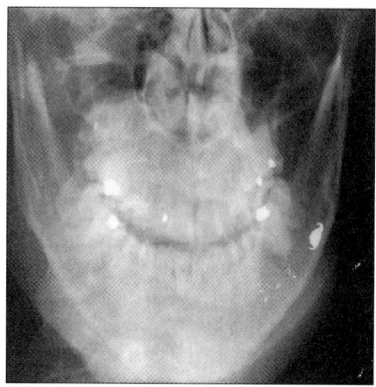

142 (a) What abnormality is shown in this postero-anterior radiograph?
(b) What other radiographic views would be necessary?
(c) What is the likely diagnosis?
(d) Outline the management.

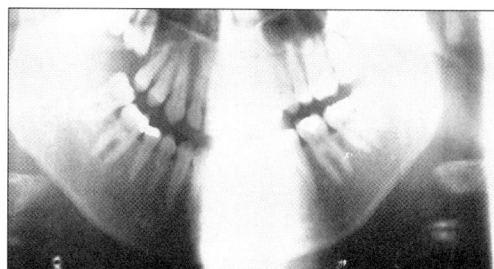

143 What errors are present on this dental panoramic tomograph?

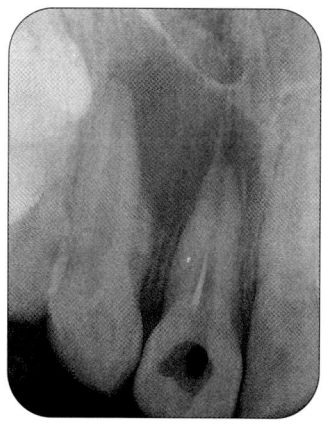

144 This patient has experienced pain from the right upper anterior region. The right upper central incisor root canal has been opened for drainage.
(a) What abnormalities are apparent on this periapical radiograph?
(b) What further treatment is needed?

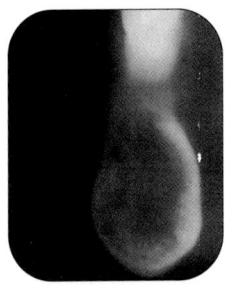

145 (a) What is the radiographic view shown?
(b) Describe the appearance illustrated.
(c) What is the most likely diagnosis?

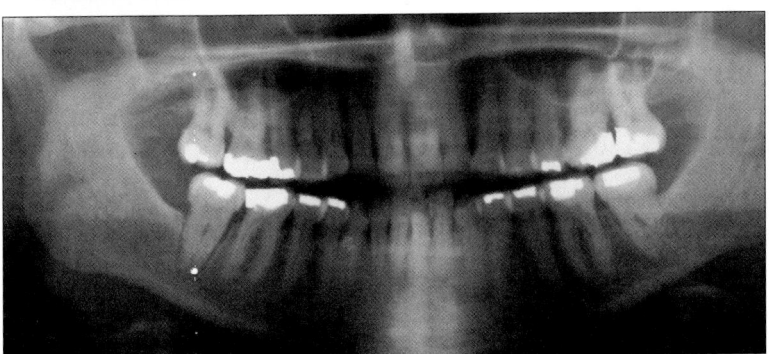

146 This 40-year-old woman presents with increasing difficulty in opening her mouth. There is no facial swelling or discomfort, but a reduced laxity of her cheeks and lips. None of her teeth are loose or tender to percussion. The dental panoramic radiograph shows widening of the periodontal ligament space around 5̲and 7̲6̲7̲.
(a) What is the most likely diagnosis?
(b) What other features may be present in patients with this condition?
(c) What other conditions may cause widening of the periodontal ligament space?

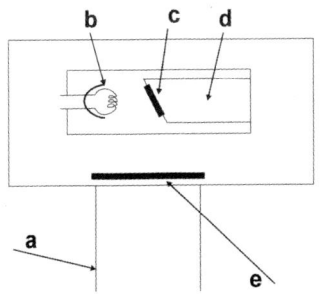

147 (a) Identify **a–e** in this diagram of a stationary anode dental X-ray tube-head.
(b) From what material is **c** constructed and why?
(c) What is the effect of increasing the kilovoltage of the X-ray set?

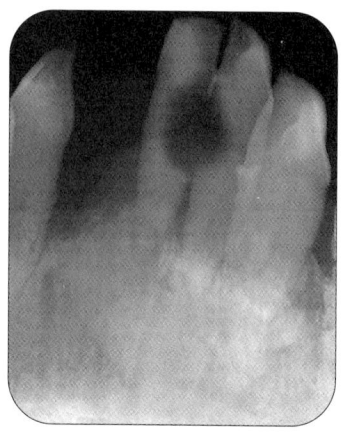

148 (a) What is the diagnosis of the radiolucent lesions present on ⊤2 in this periapical radiograph?
(b) What is the cause of the linear radiolucencies seen running vertically in the bone?

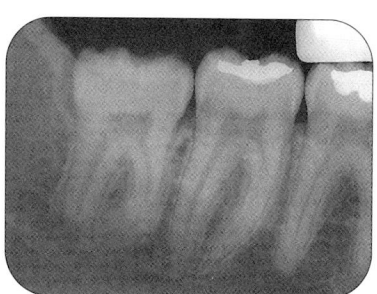

149 (a) Describe the radiological assessment of the unerupted lower right wisdom tooth illustrated in this periapical radiograph.
(b) Is a further radiograph required to assist with determining the positional relationship of the root to the inferior alveolar canal? If so, why and what view?

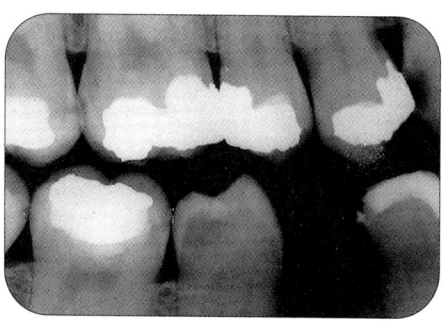

150 What do you note on this bitewing radiograph of the lower right posterior region?

1 (a) Oblique lateral radiograph of the left side of the mandible.
   (b) Other radiographic views include:
       (i) Lower true (90°) occlusal.
       (ii) Postero-anterior radiograph, centred on the jaws.
       These additional views are required to assess the degree of buccolingual expansion of the mandible caused by the lesion.
       (iii) Computerized tomography may show the full extent of the lesion within the bone, and demonstrate any extension of the lesion into the condyle and coronoid process, together with possible bony perforation and its extension into the soft tissues.
   (c) A multilocular lesion (approximately 4 x 8 cm) is situated at the angle of the left side of the mandible, extending anteriorly to the second premolar, posteriorly and superiorly as far as the coronoid process and sigmoid notch, and inferiorly to the lower border of the mandible. It is of variable radiodensity due to its multilocular nature and the differential extent of cortical bone resorption, but there is no evidence of calcification within it. The outline or edge of the lesion is well-defined and partly corticated. The roots of the related lower premolar and molar teeth are resorbed apically. The vertical height of the mandible appears increased in the retromolar region, suggesting an expanding lesion. The mediolateral expansion cannot be determined from this view.
   (d) The most likely diagnosis of an expansive, multilocular lesion at the posterior body and ramus of the mandible in this age group is an ameloblastoma. Other conditions that would need to be considered in a radiological differential diagnosis include: an odontogenic keratocyst, odontogenic myxoma, odontogenic fibroma, and giant cell lesions, such as central giant cell granuloma, aneurysmal bone cyst, and brown tumour of hyperparathyroidism (although there is no other radiographic evidence of hyperparathyroidism). The ameloblastoma and the myxoma tend to cause root resorption.
       Histological examination revealed the lesion to be an ameloblastoma. Treatment, in general, involves excision of the lesion with a margin of normal bone; thus, large tumours may require resection of the mandible.

2 (a) A gutta percha point that has been passed along the sinus tract as an aid to diagnosis. Note that it is of similar density to the material in the root canal of the incisor.
   (b) The root is shorter than normal, having an incompletely formed root canal which is wider than normal and has an open apex. This appearance suggests the probability of trauma, at an approximate age of 8–10 years, resulting in pulp necrosis and premature arrest of root development.
   (c) The periapical radiolucency together with the presence of a sinus are indicative of a chronic apical abscess. The tooth has an open apex and an inadequately condensed root filling. An orthograde root canal filling should be attempted, but in view of the shape and size of the root canal, a paste dressing, such as a calcium hydroxide based material, would be preferable. Once an apical barrier has been obtained, then a permanent root filling can be placed.

ANSWERS

3 (a) Most of the teeth show enlarged pulp chambers which are particularly clearly seen in the lower primary molars. There is also extensive alveolar bone loss, mainly affecting the upper primary incisors.

(b) The condition is childhood hypophosphatasia. Hypophosphatasia is an inherited disorder characterized by a deficiency in serum alkaline phosphatase in conjunction with defective mineralization of the skeletal and dental structures. Four types are described – perinatal/lethal, infantile, childhood, and adult hypophosphatasia, with survival to adulthood only likely in the last two forms. In the childhood form, cemental aplasia/hypoplasia results in early primary tooth loss, mainly affecting the incisor teeth. There is horizontal alveolar bone loss resulting from disuse atrophy, as there is no mechanical stimulation of the bone through the fibres of the periodontal ligament, due to the absence of cementum. Consequently, the teeth exfoliate. The adult form is usually diagnosed during middle age and is mild, with periodontal abnormalities particularly confined to the anterior teeth. The mode of inheritance of hypophosphatasia is uncertain, with evidence for both autosomal recessive and dominant forms.

(c) In the jaws there may be a generalized radiolucency and thinning of the cortical bone and lamina dura. The calvarium may show a 'beaten copper' appearance. Radiographs of the long bones may show tongue-shaped radiolucent projections from the epiphyseal plates into the metaphases.

4 (a) The radiograph shows a number of abnormalities including:
(i) Coarse bony trabeculae enclosing the marrow spaces in the mandible, maxilla, and zygoma.
(ii) Generalized loss of the lamina dura.
(iii) Increase in the depth of the mandible.
(iv) Thinning of the inferior cortical plate of the mandible.
(v) Loss of the outline of the inferior alveolar canals.
(vi) Small maxillary sinuses.

(b) These features are consistent with a bone marrow replacement disorder, in this example, thalassaemia intermedia. The patient has a haemoglobin of 10 g/l, which suggests that the features have arisen from compensatory hyperplasia of the haematopoietic tissue throughout the jaws, resulting in enlargement of the marrow spaces. Patients with thalassaemia minor or major rarely demonstrate significant radiographic features, the latter because they are usually receiving regular blood transfusions as part of their management.

5 (a) Lower joint space TMJ arthrogram (single contrast). Variations on this technique include dual joint space arthrography, where contrast is also introduced into the superior joint space, and double-contrast arthrography, where air is introduced into the same space in addition to the contrast medium.

(b) Imaging of the disc and other soft tissues of the TMJ is indicated when there is a suspected internal derangement of the joint, in a patient whose symptoms have been unresponsive to conservative treatment and in whom complex or invasive treatment (e.g. open surgery) is being considered. Magnetic resonance imaging

(MRI) is increasingly used instead of arthrography, as it is non-invasive, but the images may not provide the fine detail of arthrograms. Both arthrography and MRI require skilful technique and interpretation.

(c) There are two main contra-indications to the use of this technique:

(i) Hypersensitivity. Patients may be hypersensitive to iodine or, possibly, other components of the contrast medium. A history of previous reactions may be elicited.

(ii) The presence of local infection, either of the joint (infective arthritis) or of other nearby structures (e.g., otitis externa).

(d) The view taken with the mouth closed shows radiopaque contrast medium in the lower joint space of the TMJ; the needle through which medium was injected is also evident. A large collection of medium extends well anterior to the head of the condyle. This appearance is consistent with a disc which is markedly displaced anteriorly. The 'fully open' view shows that the condyle has translated slightly anteriorly, but that the contrast pattern is unchanged; this indicates that the disc has failed to reduce into a normal position. Such an anteriorly displaced disc may interfere with full condylar movement.

6 (a) A computerized tomograph (CT) showing a slice in an axial plane at the level of the first cervical vertebra. This technique has the advantage of demonstrating both bone and soft tissue structures.

(b) There is a relatively high attenuation (appears as a lighter shade of grey) mass within the right parotid gland, posterolateral to the ramus of the mandible. This gland usually has a low attenuation (dark) appearance (see the left parotid gland) due to the presence of fat within it, which increases with age, enhancing the differentiation of the tumour, which has an appearance similar to that of muscle (see illustration).

(c) A pleomorphic salivary adenoma, which is the most common neoplasm of the parotid gland. It most often occurs in middle-aged women and presents as a slowly enlarging mass just anterior to the pinna of the ear. Weakness of the muscles of facial expression is not a typical feature of this condition, because pleomorphic adenomas are generally benign and thus displace, rather than infiltrate, those branches of the facial nerve which traverse the parotid gland.

(d) (i) Diagnostic ultrasound is a useful technique for the initial investigation of a soft tissue mass, to confirm its presence, consistency, and size. It is relatively inexpensive, widely available, and does not involve exposure to ionizing radiation.

(ii) Magnetic resonance imaging also does not involve irradiation and is an alternative to CT scanning. As with CT scanning, magnetic resonance images enable the approximate position of the course of the facial nerve within the parotid gland to be determined.

(iii) Scintiscanning may demonstrate tumours as 'hot' or 'cold' spots, depending on whether they take up the radionuclide or not. However, it is a less sensitive investigation than those outlined above.

(e) Surgical removal, usually by a superficial parotidectomy for those lateral to the facial nerve or by removal of the gland for those more deeply placed. Pleomorphic adenomas are usually incompletely encapsulated and frequently have localized nodular outgrowths, so that enucleation often results in incomplete removal.

7 (a) Approximately one-third of the mesial root $\overline{7|}$ is retained, there is a smaller root fragment in the distal socket, and a few radiodense particles are present at the coronal aspect of the socket.

(b) (i) Infected socket due to retained root fragments.
(ii) Localized alveolar osteitis (dry socket).
(iii) Pulpitis or possibly early apical periodontitis $\overline{8|}$, resulting from the untreated occlusal carious lesion.
(iv) Pericoronitis associated with the impacted $\overline{8|}$. There is slight widening of the follicular space mesially.

(c) The state of the lower right second molar, prior to extraction, is unknown. However, its retained mesial root appears slender, similar to that of the roots of the lower first molar, and the alveolar bone is sclerotic. There is attrition of the crowns of all the teeth, suggesting that excessive occlusal load may have led to the bony sclerosis. This combination of narrow roots and alveolar sclerosis often predisposes to difficulty with tooth extraction.

(d) Periapical radiographs of $\overline{87|}$ would be advisable to clarify the size, shape, and position of the retained roots, the configuration of the roots of the third molar, and their relationship to the inferior alveolar canal.

(e) The radiopaque metallic object is a nose stud.

8 (a) A three-dimensional image reconstructed from a series of slices obtained by computerized tomography. The three-dimensional effect is obtained by presenting those structures lying anteriorly in a lighter shade than those more posteriorly. Once the slices have been reconstructed, the three-dimensional image may be rotated on the computer screen so that it can be viewed from different aspects. Three-dimensional reconstruction is particularly helpful in the assessment of severe facial deformity, either from developmental causes or following trauma.

(b) There is very little alveolar bone in either the maxilla or the mandible. In addition, there is a bony deficiency in the maxilla in the left anterior region due to a cleft palate.

9 (a) The trabecular pattern is very fine, producing an appearance known variously as ground glass, orange peel, or finger print. In addition, the lamina dura is not evident around the roots of the teeth. The cavity and floor of the antrum are not apparent.

(b) Three conditions that typically produce this radiographic appearance are:
(i) Fibrous dysplasia (as in this example).
(ii) Hyperparathyroidism.
(iii) Paget's disease of bone in its early stages.

(c) Other investigations include:
(i) A dental panoramic tomograph to assess the full extent of the lesion and whether other areas in the jaws are involved.

(ii) A true lateral skull radiograph to assess possible cranial vault involvement.

(iii) Serum biochemistry to assess, in particular, the levels of calcium, phosphate, alkaline phosphatase, and parathormone.

Fibrous dysplasia, hyperparathyroidism, and the early stage of Paget's disease of bone are unrelated conditions, but may have a similar radiographic appearance. Fibrous dysplasia is a localized fibro-cemento-osseous lesion that occurs mostly in children and young adults; within the lesion there is proliferation of fibrous tissue and resorption of normal bone, followed by replacement with woven bone. There is enlargement of the affected part of the jaw. Two clinical varieties exist – monostotic, which affects just one bone and is the more common type, and polyostotic, which affects more than one bone. The radiographic appearance of fibrous dysplasia varies according to the relative amounts of fibrous and osseous tissues present. In general, immature lesions are more radiolucent and sometimes have well-defined margins, while the more mature lesions are of mixed density or uniformly radiopaque with indistinct margins (as illustrated in the question). Hyperparathyroidism is a generalized disorder found more commonly in women between 40 and 60 years of age, with an incidence of approximately 1 in 1000. It is usually caused primarily by an adenoma of the parathyroid glands or secondary to kidney disease, both of which result in an increased secretion of parathormone. As a consequence, there is generalized bone resorption and a rise in the plasma calcium levels. The typical radiological features are subperiosteal erosions, particularly of the phalanges, generalized demineralization, radiolucent lesions (the so-called brown tumours), and soft tissue calcifications. In the jaws, the loss of the lamina dura is an early radiological sign. The generalized demineralization is caused by thinning of the trabeculae which, paradoxically on a radiograph, tends to produce a ground-glass appearance.

Paget's disease of bone is a disease of the elderly and tends to affect particular bones, notably the skull, vertebrae, and long bones. It is characterized in the early stages by bone resorption leading to radiolucency, most noticeably in the skull (e.g., osteoporosis circumscripta of the skull) and in the later stages by bone deposition leading to radiopacity. When either of the jaws is involved, bony changes tend to be bilateral and the affected bones show an increase in size. In the dentate, there may be a generalized partial absence of the lamina dura, the roots may exhibit hypercementosis, and there may be focal areas of sclerosis of the periapical bone.

10 (a) There is a discontinuity of the floor of the right orbit, the fragments of which have been displaced into the maxillary antrum. Through this defect some of the soft tissue contents of the orbit (fat and muscle) are also partially displaced. In addition, the lower part of the right maxillary antrum contains material of high attenuation with a horizontal upper margin, typical of a fluid level.

(b) Fracture of the orbital floor with displacement of the orbital contents into the maxillary antrum (orbital 'blow-out' fracture).

(c) The cardinal signs of this injury are:

(i) Paraesthesia of the distribution of the infra-orbital nerve (ipsilateral skin of cheek, upper labial and gingival mucosa, and upper incisors).

(ii) Enophthalmos (globe of the eye sunk into the orbit).

(iii) Restricted movements of the eye, particularly on upward gaze.

(iv) A drop in the pupillary level compared with the contralateral side.

The cardinal symptoms of the injury are:

(i) Numbness of the cheek, mucosa, and teeth.

(ii) Diplopia.

(d) The typical features in an occipitomental radiograph would include:

(i) A 'tear-drop' shaped radiopacity hanging from the orbital floor into the upper part of the maxillary antrum.

(ii) The bony outline of the inferior aspect of the orbital rim remains intact.

(iii) Opacity of the lower part of the maxillary antrum with a horizontal upper margin, indicative of fluid (in this example, blood) within the cavity.

(iv) Intra-orbital air, as shown by discrete areas of radiolucency usually seen in the superior aspect of the orbit.

11 (a) There is a loculated irregularly shaped radiolucency, which has a well-defined corticated margin anteriorly, but which is less well-defined elsewhere. Within the main radiolucency are several coarse bony trabeculae. There is slight expansion of the alveolar crest.

(b) The differential diagnosis of a loculated radiolucency containing coarse trabeculations includes:

(i) Central giant cell granuloma.

(ii) Odontogenic myxoma.

(iii) Aneurysmal bone cyst (as in this example).

The aneurysmal bone cyst usually occurs in young adults. Its aetiology is unknown, but it may be a reactive phenomenon arising within another lesion, such as a giant-cell granuloma or cemento-ossifying fibroma. Usually, it contains numbers of large, blood-filled channels. The typical radiographic appearance is of a ballooned radiolucency containing several bony trabeculae, which may represent uneven resorption of the bone. The lesion has three phases – an osteolytic phase, a growth phase in which there is rapid enlargement, and a mature stage in which growth continues and the trabeculations become more obvious. The example illustrated represents the osteolytic phase, which is less typical of the condition than the later phases. Fluid levels within the lesion may be seen on computerized tomography, particularly if the patient has been resting for a few minutes prior to examination. Treatment is by surgical removal; however, recurrence is common.

12 (a) The teeth have bulbous crowns and short 'spiky' roots, an appearance that is found in many dentine and pulp dysplasias. However, this patient has relatively normal dentine formation. This condition is a generalized short-root anomaly.

(b) Short-rooted teeth may be associated with several generalized conditions, including endocrine disorders such as hypoparathyroidism, tumoral calcinosis,

Ellis-van Creveld syndrome, and hemi-facial hypoplasia. There is often a familial pattern in patients with this condition and racial variations are recognized, with shorter roots generally being found in people of mongoloid origin.

The patient shown here had a very short stature – 99 cm at the age of 17 years – and some unusual skeletal abnormalities. This combination of short stature and generalized short-root anomaly is unusual.

13 (a) Although the periapical radiographic views have not been standardized, it is clear that there has been a significant amount of alveolar bone loss affecting 1⌋. The bone resorption between 1⌋1 in **13A** is mainly horizontal and has involved the coronal one-third of the roots. In **13B**, there has been much further bone resorption, especially affecting the mesial root surface , which appears to have occurred in the absence of local factors, such as overhanging restorations and subgingival calculus. In addition, there is widening of the periodontal ligament space distally 1⌋ suggesting that this tooth may exhibit some increase in mobility.

(b) Rapidly progressing periodontitis (generalized early onset periodontitis). Although the lesion involves an incisor tooth, more typical of juvenile periodontitis (localized early onset periodontitis), the age of the patient largely excludes that diagnosis.

(c) Assuming that the patient wishes to save the teeth:
(i) Check on the vitality of the upper incisor teeth.
(ii) If vital, decontaminate the root surfaces with a localized antibacterial agent, such as metronidazole, followed by root planing. If this treatment is unsuccessful, consider flap surgery with or without guided tissue regeneration.
(iii) If the tooth is non-vital, in addition it will require root canal therapy.

14 (a) There is an oval, well-defined radiolucency, approximately 15 mm in diameter, distal to and partly overlying the distal root and part of the crown of ⎺8 . It does not extend as far as the apex of this tooth, which is caries free. The lamina dura distally ⎺8 is absent. The alveolar bone crest height is normal.

(b) Paradental cyst, thought to be inflammatory in origin, due to stimulation of the reduced enamel epithelium or the cell rests of Malassez. The cyst most commonly develops on the buccal aspect of a partially erupted lower third molar. In virtually all cases there is a history of pericoronitis, often recurrent in nature. Treatment involves removal of the tooth and the cyst.

15 (a) There is moderate periodontal bone loss around all of the teeth shown, involving approximately the coronal one-third of the root. The bone loss appears more advanced on the mesial aspect of the root of ⎺7⌋, but its extent has been exaggerated because this tooth is tilted mesially. There is, however, a small area of radiolucency in the root bifurcation, indicating early bone loss at this site. There is occlusal caries present on 5⌋, which has extended to involve the dentine.

(b) The full extent of the bone loss is not completely demonstrated, thus periapical radiographs taken with the paralleling technique or vertical bitewing radiographs are required. It is probable that the teeth in the other quadrants of the mouth are similarly affected, so a full mouth radiographic examination is indicated.

(c) The tilting of $\overline{7|}$ and the closure of the space between $\overline{7|}$ and $\overline{5|}$ has resulted in an area of stagnation, which has favoured the accumulation of dental plaque.

16 (a) There is a generalized lack of radiodensity of the mandible, particularly noticeable in the cortical bone, which appears thinner than normal. In addition, it is difficult to delineate the laminae of the inferior alveolar canal. The trabeculae within the cancellous bone appear thinner and fewer than normal, to give a somewhat uniform granular radiodensity. A similar appearance is seen to affect the cervical vertebrae.

(b) Osteoporosis, defined as a deficiency of bone tissue per unit volume. The bone trabeculae are histologically normal, but radiographically the bones appear less dense. It is a feature of ageing, being most pronounced in postmenopausal women. However, it can occur, for example, in malnutrition, uncontrolled diabetes, and with prolonged administration of certain drugs, such as corticosteroids. When osteoporosis affects other bones it has serious consequences, such as vertebral collapse and fracture of the neck of the femur.

17 (a) The main radiographic changes evident in the cranial vault and jaws include:
(i) Bone resorption in the anterior half of the cranium, with a scalloped posterior margin, described as osteoporosis circumscripta. The occipital region appears normal.
(ii) Haphazard foci of bone deposition in the frontal region of the cranium causing thickening of the bone, which may progress to cause enlargement of the skull. These foci are described as resembling cotton wool patches.
(iii) Increased deposition of bone in the alveolar part of the maxilla showing a similar cotton wool appearance.

(b) The patient may complain that his upper jaw appears to be getting larger and that his upper denture no longer fits properly. He may also complain of bone pain. Coincidentally, the patient may also mention that his hats seem to be getting tighter or no longer fit.

(c) Paget's disease of bone, a disease of unknown cause that affects the elderly, in which the balance between the normal processes of bone deposition and resorption is disturbed. Bones commonly involved include the calvarium, one or both of the jaws, and the stress-bearing long bones. The involvement of the skull is particularly characteristic. Initially, there are areas of radiolucency starting anteriorly and spreading posteriorly towards the occipital region, an appearance described as osteoporosis circumscripta. Later, the bones of the skull increase in thickness and their shape distorts resulting in basillar invagination, the so-called 'tam-o'-shanter' appearance. In the jaws an early radiographic feature is a ground-glass appearance (see **9**), later developing into cotton wool patches as the haphazard deposition of bone becomes predominant. Involvement of the stress-bearing long bones can result in softening and bending, so accounting for the other name of this condition, osteitis deformans. The condition is accompanied by an increase, often marked, in the serum alkaline phosphatase levels.

18   Three possible ways are shown in the table below – comparing it with the effective dose from other radiographic examinations, with the risk of death from radiation-induced cancer and with the equivalent exposure to natural background radiation.

	Effective dose (mSv)	Risk of fatal cancer/10^6 examinations	Equivalent natural background radiation
2 bitewing radiographs, 70kV, 20 cm fsd*, rectangular collimation, E-speed film	0.002	0.1	8 hr
A skull radiograph	0.01	0.6	41 hr
A barium meal examination	5	300	2.3 years

* fsd = focus skin distance

19 (a) Distal, mesiolingual, and mesio-buccal root canals. In this example of a lower second molar, the mesial root has two separate root canals, one buccally and one lingually. The oblique angulation of the X-ray beam has overcome the problem of superimposition of the two files in the mesial root. It has projected the image of the file in the buccal canal, which lies closer to the tube, further mesially compared with the one in the mesiolingual root canal (see diagram).

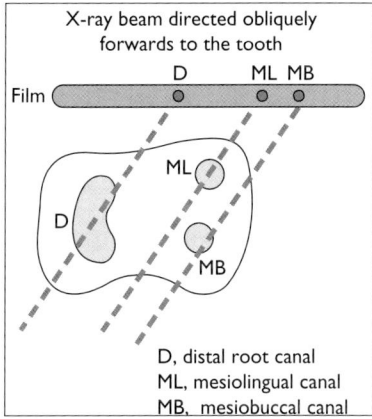

X-ray beam directed obliquely forwards to the tooth

Film

D   ML MB

ML

D

MB

D, distal root canal
ML, mesiolingual canal
MB, mesiobuccal canal

(b) The tip of a straight Spencer Wells forceps. These are convenient for holding the film when taking a radiograph in the lower posterior region of the mouth, particularly during root canal therapy, when access for film holders is restricted.

ANSWERS

20 (a) The roots of all the upper incisor teeth are shortened markedly as a consequence of root resorption. The periodontal ligament space around these teeth is widened, particularly at the apex of 2|. The apices of the other teeth are flattened and the absence of periapical radiolucencies suggests that the resorption is no longer active. There is alveolar bone loss at the interdental crests due to chronic adult periodontitis. This combination of effects (bone loss and root resorption) has resulted in increased mobility of the teeth, as indicated by the widening of the periodontal ligament spaces. The condition has been managed by the application of a splint composed of stainless steel wires embedded in composite. There are multiple interstitial radiolucent restorations and an amalgam restoration,|1 .

(b) (i) Excessive parafunctional tooth contacts.
(ii) Use of excessive force during orthodontic tooth movement (as in this example).
(iii) Idiopathic root resorption.

(c) (i) Regular, 3-monthly, review appointments to ensure that there is a high standard of oral hygiene, in order to minimize further periodontal bone loss.
(ii) Appropriate radiographic review. In this example this was initially carried out at 24-monthly intervals, to check for the presence of possible further resorption.

21 (a) Approximately 9–10 years old, as determined from the stages of eruption and root development of the lateral and central incisors.

(b) There is a horizontal mid-root fracture with displacement of the coronal fragment and slight widening of the periodontal ligament at the fracture site. The pulp in the apical root fragment is likely to be vital as there is evidence of continuing normal root development since the accident. Therefore, no treatment other than regular clinical and radiographic review is required at present.

22 (a) The most striking feature is the grossly enlarged left mandibular condyle. Its margins are well defined, but a little irregular. There is lengthening of the left ramus, a 'bowing' of the left mandibular angle and lower border, and a left posterior open bite. There is also a relatively small coronoid process on the left.

(b) The most likely diagnosis is a hyperplasia of the left mandibular condyle. The overactivity of the condylar cartilage usually arises during the normal growth phase of the individual and stops or slows down after body growth ceases. The differential diagnosis should include a neoplasm, such as an osteochondroma, although these usually appear as a more localized mass attached to the condyle.

23 (a) (i) *Upper left quadrant:* One premolar is missing, the other, probably the first premolar, is grossly decayed, and has been root-treated but has a periapical radiolucency. The first molar has a large amalgam restoration. One root canal of the second molar has been treated endodontically and the tooth bears a pin-retained restoration; again, there is a periapical radiolucency. The third molar is unopposed and slightly overerupted.

(ii) *Lower left quadrant:* The first molar has been root-treated and there is extensive caries with loss of the crown. There is a periapical radiolucency involving both apices, suggestive of a granuloma. The second molar has a large occlusal amalgam restoration and the third molar is unerupted and transversely impacted. (iii) *Lower right quadrant:* The healing of the tooth socket of the first molar, which was extracted a few months previously, is well advanced. The second molar has an amalgam restoration. The third molar is horizontally impacted and grossly carious.

(iv) *Upper right quadrant:* The second premolar has been root-treated and the crown is absent. The second molar has also been root-treated and bears a pin-retained porcelain jacket crown. The third molar has an amalgam restoration and is overerupted. The first premolar and first molar also have amalgam restorations.

(b) These findings suggest a history of extensive restorative dental treatment, in a patient who is prone to dental caries. There appears to have been a phase of neglect with recurrent caries, loss of the crowns of some teeth, development of periapical lesions, and a relatively recent tooth extraction.

(c) A lower true (90%) occlusal radiograph would be necessary to demonstrate the buccolingual orientation of $\overline{8}$.

(d) This is a metallic structure, either a necklace or a dental bib chain.

24 (a) A ventriculoperitoneal shunt placed in the ventricles of the brain for drainage of cerebrospinal fluid into the peritoneal cavity.

(b) Such shunts are inserted to treat patients who suffer from hydrocephalus. Hydrocephalus arises from an imbalance between the production and absorption of cerebrospinal fluid, resulting in a raised intracranial pressure and an enlargement of the ventricular system. If left untreated it leads to enlargement of the cranium and may also result in spasticity, ataxia, and progressive mental deterioration. The ventriculoperitoneal shunt contains a one-way valve to allow discharge of excessive cerebrospinal fluid from the ventricular system.

(c) Apart from any difficulties in the management of patients with spasticity or learning difficulties, there are also problems associated with the shunt itself. These, in common with other similar catheters, provide a potential nidus for bacterial colonization and so predispose the patient to recurrent episodes of septicaemia and ventriculitis. There have been reports of such infections following dental procedures, although there is controversy over whether antibiotic prophylaxis is required for dental procedures that result in bacteraemia. However, many paediatric neurosurgeons and neurologists recommend such prophylaxis.

25 (a) Postero-anterior radiograph centred on the jaws.

(b) The patient is positioned facing the film with the head tilted forwards, so that the radiographic baseline (the line extending from the outer canthus of the eye to the external auditory meatus) is horizontal and at right angles to the film – the so-called forehead–nose position. The X-ray beam is also horizontal and centred through the rami of the mandible.

(c) A dental panoramic tomograph or right and left oblique lateral radiographs of the mandible. Either of these views would provide an image at right angles to that of the radiograph illustrated.

(d) The radiograph shows bilateral well-defined, corticated, multilocular radiolucent lesions occupying the posterior body, angle, and ascending rami of the mandible and causing medial and lateral expansion. It is not possible from this one view to ascertain what effect the lesions are having on the nearby teeth.

(e) The most likely diagnosis is cherubism, a rare giant cell lesion of the jaws affecting young children. It is usually inherited as an autosomal dominant, although some cases may occur spontaneously. The disease is characterized by large expansile giant cell lesions affecting both sides of either the mandible or the maxilla. The lesions can cause marked enlargement and distortion of the normal facial contour. The term cherubism was introduced because, in addition to the chubby cheeks, the gross bilateral enlargement of the maxillae make it seem that the children's eyes look upwards or heavenwards. Often the teeth in the affected areas are displaced and/or delayed in eruption. Management involves biopsy, for confirmation of the diagnosis, and reassurance of the family, as growth of these lesions slows down when puberty is reached. Growth is followed by slow regression until by middle age a normal facial contour may be restored, although the radiographic appearance may still be abnormal. Sometimes, if the facial appearance is unacceptable, surgical curettage or paring down of excessive tissue may be attempted.

26 (a) There is a densely radiopaque mass lying distal to $\underline{2|}$. It contains a number of separate, small tooth-like structures (denticles) and is surrounded by a thin radiolucent capsular space, beyond which is a rim of cortical bone. $\underline{C|}$, which is retained, has only a small amount of root remaining, $\underline{3|}$ is unerupted and displaced distally, and there is no resorption of $\underline{2|}$.

(b) A compound odontome. This is a harmatomatous lesion of dental tissues in which there is a relatively ordered arrangement of enamel, dentine, cementum, and pulpal tissues into small discrete tooth-like structures. It is most commonly found in the anterior aspect of the maxilla, where it may interfere with the eruption of an adjacent tooth. Initially, before mineralization, it appears as a radiolucency when a definitive radiographic diagnosis is more difficult.

(c) In this case surgical removal of the odontome is indicated, together with the exposure of $\underline{3|}$ to allow its eruption. Orthodontic traction and alignment may be required.

27 (a) There are interstitial radiolucent lesions present mesially $\underline{|4}$, distally $\underline{|5}$, and mesially $\underline{|6}$, which appear to be centred on the enamel–cement junction. They have extended some considerable distance into the dentine to undermine the enamel, and encroach upon the pulp chambers. The radiolucencies are well defined with a 'punched out' appearance; within that involving $\underline{|4}$ there are some irregular radiopacities. The tip of the alveolar crest between $\underline{|6}$ and $\underline{|5}$ is radiolucent, with loss of the lamina dura distally $\underline{|5}$ and mesially $\underline{|4}$.

(b) Idiopathic external root resorption. Excluding the normal shedding of the primary dentition, root resorption may be caused by a number of factors, including:
(i) Chronic inflammation (e.g., periapical granuloma).

(ii) Prolonged application of excessive force (e.g., orthodontic traction).

(iii) Reimplantation or transplantation of a tooth.

(iv) Direct pressure from an enlarging tumour (e.g., ameloblastoma) or cyst.

However, in many cases the cause is unknown (idiopathic), as in this example.

Root resorption usually starts on the outer tooth surface (external) and very occasionally from the pulpodentinal aspect (internal). The enamel surface of unerupted teeth is protected by the reduced enamel epithelium and so does not usually undergo resorption, unless this layer breaks down. However, occasionally an unerupted tooth may show generalized resorption. This occurs more often with a tooth in the maxilla, particularly if it has been buried for a considerable time.

28 (a) There is a well-defined, unilocular, largely corticated radiolucency in the maxilla between 4| and |4, extending from the alveolar crest to the floor of the nose. Scattered throughout the radiolucency are numerous small irregularly shaped radiopaque foci. The lesion is partly superimposed over the crown and root of 3, which is displaced and tilted distally. The apex of the root of C|is slightly resorbed.

(b) Adenomatoid odontogenic tumour. Typically, this lesion:

(i) Is diagnosed in the second decade of life.

(ii) Occurs more often in women than men.

(iii) Occurs in the anterior part of the jaws, being found in the maxilla more often than in the mandible.

(iv) Is associated with an unerupted tooth.

(v) Contains numerous flecks of mineralization.

The adenomatoid odontogenic tumour is either a harmatoma or a benign neoplasm derived from enamel epithelium. Although it most often occurs during the second decade of life, it may be diagnosed in older individuals.

Radiographic features are of a well-defined unilocular radiolucency, frequently associated with an unerupted tooth, which contains radiopacities randomly distributed or focally arranged. These features, when present (as in this example), strongly support the diagnosis of adenomatoid odontogenic tumour. Some lesions, however, contain very few or no discernible radiopacities, when they may resemble a dentigerous cyst. Other pericoronal radiolucencies that contain radiopacities include calcifying odontogenic cysts and calcifying epithelial odontogenic tumours; however, these are usually found in people over 40 years of age. Ameloblastic fibro-odontomes (see **135**) do occur in the young, but are usually located to the posterior regions of the jaws.

(c) The adenomatoid odontogenic tumour is treated by enucleation; recurrence is uncommon.

29 (a) A lower true (90°) occlusal radiograph.

(b) There is an irregularly shaped radiopacity, approximately 6 mm in diameter, lingually to the mandible in the lower right premolar region, which shows some evidence of concentric laminations.

(c) A stone (sialolith) in the anterior part of the submandibular duct.

(d) This condition may present in one of several ways:

(i) Typically, there is recurrent pain and swelling of short duration of the associated gland when eating.

(ii) Progressive and persistent swelling of the gland caused by chronic obstructive sialadenitis.

(iii) Acute inflammatory episodes resulting in acute swelling of the affected gland and the floor of the mouth, marked pain and tenderness on palpation, and a discharge of pus from the duct orifice. These episodes of acute sialadenitis are a consequence of reduced salivary flow caused by acinar atrophy in the inflamed gland.

(iv) Sometimes the patient is symptomless and the stone is detected as an incidental radiographic finding. Paradoxically, this is more common with larger stones which may obstruct the duct less completely.

30 (a) There is a well-defined radiolucency situated distal to and partly overlying the crown of the unerupted $\overline{7|}$, which has displaced the unerupted 8| distosuperiorly. A V-shaped (with the apex pointing mesially) radiolucent fracture line extends anteriorly from the inferior border of the mandible in the molar region and loops posteriorly to cross the apical part of the roots $\overline{7|}$ into the radiolucent lesion.

(b) A fracture of the right body of the mandible. The fracture involves the cystic lesion (most likely a dentigerous cyst) associated with the crown 7|. The cyst was present prior to the accident and had caused a localized weakness of the mandible, predisposing it to fracture.

31 (a) Salivary gland scintiscan.

(b) A radionuclide which is selectively metabolized by the salivary glands is administered intravenously. The substance most commonly used is technetium pertechnetate, which is concentrated and excreted by the salivary gland ducts and also metabolized by the thyroid gland. Technetium in its metastable form emits gamma rays and the amount of radioactivity emitted by the gland is a function of acinar activity. The radionuclide appears in the ducts within 2–3 minutes, with further concentration over the next 30–40 minutes. The amount of radiation emitted by the glands is measured and displayed on a television monitor; also, it may be stored as a permanent image for future reference.

(c) There is virtually no activity in either of the parotid glands and only a small amount of uptake in the submandibular salivary glands. The thyroid gland, however, shows normal activity (this organ is clearly visible as a bilobed structure at the bottom of the image).

(d) Sjögren's syndrome.

(e) Sjögren's syndrome is usually classified into primary and secondary forms. In the former, in addition to xerostomia the patient has xerophthalmia (dry eyes). In secondary Sjögren's syndrome there is also some form of connective tissue disease, most commonly rheumatoid arthritis. The reduction in the amount of saliva may predispose to difficulty with mastication and swallowing and to an overgrowth of oral flora. This in turn may lead to increased dental caries rates, salivary gland infections, and mucosal infections, most notably candidosis. There is also an increased risk of malignant lymphoma, both in the salivary glands and in other lymphoid tissues.

(f) Management is aimed at easing the patient's symptoms and includes the use of artificial saliva and tears, scrupulous oral hygiene, and regular dental follow-up.

32 The procedures, which are set out in the *Local Rules* pertaining to a particular working environment, include:

(a) Switch off the X-ray set and disconnect it from the mains supply.

(b) Undertake a preliminary investigation to determine the probable cause and duration of the exposure.

(c) If it is likely that the patient has received at least 20 times 'normal' exposure, inform the Health & Safety Executive who may wish to carry out a detailed examination.

(d) Do not use the X-ray set again until the fault has been identified and corrected by an appropriately trained engineer.

(e) All the records associated with the incident should be kept for 50 years.

33 (a) Florid cemento-osseous dysplasia (gigantiform cementoma), which typically affects middle-aged African women and appears as multiple radiolucencies, radiopacities, or mixed density lesions, often in all four posterior quadrants. These masses arise within the alveolar parts of the jaws, often, when the teeth are present, in a periapical position. In this case, the teeth in three quadrants have been extracted, but the multiple radiopacities are still evident. In the early stages, when the lesions are composed predominantly of fibrous tissue, they are radiolucent, but become progressively radiopaque as mineralized matrix is deposited. At this stage they are usually surrounded by a thin radiolucent capsule and corticated bone margin. The upper left quadrant shows that expansion and enlargement of the affected alveolar process can occur.

(b) Following extraction of the tooth the cementoma has become exposed to the oral environment and consequently become infected. Infection is more likely to occur in mature lesions which, because of their dense structure, have a poor blood supply.

34 (a) There is an irregularly shaped radiopaque mass on the right side, partly overlying the lower aspect of the mandible, but mainly situated below, just anterior to the angle.

(b) Calcification within the submandibular salivary gland. A similar appearance may be produced by calcification in a deep cervical lymph node following a chronic infection, such as tuberculosis (see **116**) . However, the position of the lesion illustrated is anterior to the cervical chain .

(c) Part of the epiglottis.

ANSWERS

35 (a) Mesial root resection, together with filling of the distal root canal and restoration with a post-retained full veneer crown.

(b) (i) Lateral perforation of the canal or fracture of the filled root. This is more likely to happen when the root is flattened mesiodistally. In this example the post is large in cross-section relative to the root, but there is no perforation.

(ii) The contour of the crown that remains after root resection may lead to difficulties in the application of routine oral hygiene procedures to the tooth and its supporting tissues.

(iii) Removal of one root from a multirooted tooth reduces the area of the bone surface to which normal occlusal forces are transmitted, so there may be functional overload, which consequently may result in increased tooth mobility, tipping, and/or fracture of the remaining root(s). This risk can be lowered by reducing the occlusal surface area of the tooth, e.g., by premolarization of the crown restoration.

36 (a) All of the teeth are much smaller than normal (microdontia) and many of them have very short roots, due to advanced resorption, with the exception of the second and third molars. The pulp chambers and root canals of most of the teeth are poorly displayed due to extensive pulpal obliteration.

(b) Variations in size of the dentition are largely of genetic origin, but also occur in some endocrine disorders. This patient has hypopituitarism, with short stature (pituitary dwarfism), and failure of sexual development. There is a discrepancy between his chronological age and his height and skeletal maturity. Hypopituitarism may also be associated with delayed exfoliation of the primary teeth and delayed eruption of the permanent teeth. Hypothyroidism may also cause a diminution in the size of the dentition, together with other dental anomalies, but it usually causes an overall delay in the development, rather than structural abnormalities of the teeth themselves.

(c) Treatment is indicated because the patient was concerned about his appearance and had some difficulty with masticatory function. Management consists of removal of the mobile anterior teeth and construction of full upper and lower overdentures.

37 (a) Osseointegration has taken place as there is no evidence of a fine radiolucent line between the threads of the implant and the adjacent alveolar bone. The titanium and bone appear to be in intimate contact.

(b) A radiograph should be taken at this stage to ensure that the abutment is fully seated against the implant fixture.

(c) A periapical radiograph provides the essential detail. It is important to use a paralleling technique with the central ray directed through the junction of the implant and the abutment.

(d) The flap should not be closed as the abutment is not fully seated down onto the implant. Compare this radiograph, which now shows the same abutment completely seated, with the one in the question.

38 (a) Transcranial oblique lateral radiographs of the right and left TMJs in the 'closed' position. During the investigation of TMJs, similar views are also frequently taken in the 'open' position.

(b) Typically, (see diagram) the patient's head is positioned with the interpupillary line at right angles to, and the mid-sagittal plane parallel to, the film. The X-ray tube is angled 25° caudally and 20° anteriorly on the contralateral side, so that the centre of the beam passes through the joint adjacent to the film.

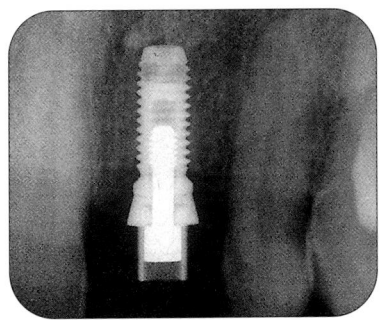

(c) These radiographs show an oblique view of the TMJ in which the following anatomical features are usually displayed:

(i) The outline and internal structure of the articular aspect of the head of the condyle, particularly its lateral side, as the image of the medial part is often obscured by superimposition of other bony structures.

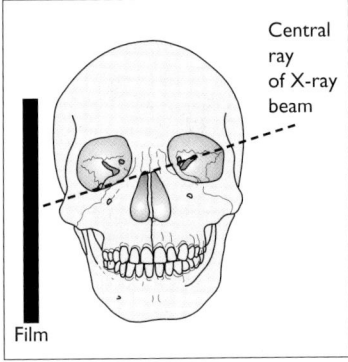

(ii) The outline of the inferior surface of the glenoid fossa.

(iii) The amount of space that is present between the lateral part of the head of the condyle and the glenoid fossa.

(d) The left TMJ (**38B**) is normal, the condylar head is of normal outline and density, and there is no narrowing of the joint space. On the other hand, the head of the right condyle (**38A**) is flattened due to resorption and bone remodelling, with compensatory osteogenesis to produce a 'beak' or 'spike' of new bone anteriorly, where there is also some sclerosis. The bone around the glenoid fossa shows sclerosis when compared with the normal side. There is narrowing of the joint space anterosuperiorly. These features are characteristic of osteoarthrosis.

A number of other radiographic changes may be observed in disorders of the TMJ. Erosion, seen either as a loss of the surface cortical bone or as a discrete radiolucency within the bone, may occur in any form of active arthritis, including rheumatoid, psoriatic, and infective disease, or secondarily to an internal disc derangement. In rheumatoid arthritis, erosion can be particularly marked, such that in advanced stages of the disease the condyle may change in shape to that of a 'sharpened pencil'. The size of the joint space may appear enlarged in several conditions, such as might occur after trauma due to a joint effusion. However, great care is required in interpreting the size of the joint space, as this can vary significantly according to the angle of the X-ray beam.

39 (a) There is a large radiolucent area in the anterior part of the maxilla. It is ovoid, with a well-defined, corticated margin, and extends from 4|to|5 , posteriorly into the hard palate, and superiorly into the floor of the nose and the maxillary antrum on the left side 3| has been displaced and tilted.
(b) The overall shape and outline suggest a benign lesion, most probably a cyst. The diagnoses therefore include:
(i) Residual cyst – the absence of |2 would support this diagnosis.
(ii) Radicular cyst – |2 is root-filled with its apex associated with the lesion, making the diagnosis of a radicular cyst a possibility, although the eccentric position of the tooth relative to the cyst and the large size of the cyst make this a less likely diagnosis.
(iii) Nasopalatine cyst – with a cystic lesion in the anterior midline of the maxilla, the diagnosis of nasopalatine cyst should always be considered.
(iv) Odontogenic keratocyst – the ovoid shape of the lesion raises the possibility of a diagnosis of odontogenic keratocyst.
The final diagnosis was a residual cyst.
(c) The main clinical features include expansion of the alveolar bone buccally and palatally. The bone may be markedly thinned or perforated, so that on palpation there would be 'eggshell crackling' or fluctuation, respectively. There would also be displacement of|3 , which may exhibit some mobility.
(d) The diagnosis could be aided by aspiration of the cyst contents and biopsy of the lining. Analysis of the cyst contents would help to differentiate preoperatively between an odontogenic keratocyst and other types of cyst. In view of the benign appearance of the lesion, incisional biopsy may be unnecessary.
(e) Periapical radiographs would demonstrate the relationship of the cyst to the teeth more clearly. Lateral and postero-anterior views of the facial bones would show the degree of vertical bone loss and provide further guidance as to the dimensions of the lesion.
(f) The cyst should be enucleated. Some of the adjacent teeth may have to be extracted due to poor bony support. Follow-up radiographs, initially at 6-month intervals, would provide an assessment of bone regeneration.

40 **1**, Zygomatic arch; **2**, pterygomaxillary fissure; **3**, medial wall of the maxillary antrum/lateral wall of the nose; **4**, inferior alveolar canal; **5**, valecula; **6**, mental foramen; **7**, epiglottis.

41 (a) A collimated oblique lateral radiograph of the body of the left side of the mandible (**41A**) and part of a lower true (90°) occlusal radiograph centred on the left premolar region (**41B**).
(b) The lesion is of mixed radiodensity – essentially a unilocular area of radiolucency containing zones of patchy radiopacity. The outline is smooth, reasonably well-defined, and corticated. The lesion has expanded the mandible buccally as well

as causing displacement of the inferior alveolar canal. The lower left second premolar and first molar are missing, presumably due to previous extraction.

(c) Cemento-ossifying fibroma is the most likely diagnosis of an expansive lesion of variable radiodensity in this age group. At one time, ossifying and cementifying fibromas were classified separately, but they are now regarded as different forms of the same lesion, hence the all-embracing term cemento-ossifying fibroma. As the name implies, it is classified as a benign neoplasm and is one of the group of fibro-cemento-osseous lesions. As with most of these lesions, cemento-ossifying fibromas are radiolucent in the early stages, during which normal bone is replaced by fibrous tissue, but in the later stages they become increasingly radiopaque as deposition of mineralized matrix occurs. The radiopaque zones eventually coalesce to form a densely radiopaque mass. The case illustrated is at an intermediate stage. Associated teeth are often displaced and may be resorbed (which may explain the early extractions in this case). The expansive nature is a typical feature of this lesion. Fibrous dysplasia occurs in a similar age group and may have a similar radiological appearance, but the margin is usually less well-defined from the surrounding bone. Cemento-ossifying fibromas are treated by surgical excision.

42 (a) Static electrical discharge.

(b) Under certain conditions there is a build-up of static electricity around the radiographic film. Upon its discharge, the energy is released in the form of tracks of electricity or flashes of visible light which result in exposure of the emulsion. Two patterns of radiolucent artefact are recognized – one in the form of branching lines emanating from a point of origin (as in this example), and the other as ill-defined circular areas of varying size. The build-up of static electricity is associated with rapid sliding movements, such as might occur when a screen film is removed from its packaging or from the pouch of a flexible cassette. It is more likely to occur in a warm dry environment and when wearing rubber gloves.

43 The $\overline{7}$ has a combined periodontal–periapical lesion involving the distobuccal root, as illustrated by the radiolucency extending along the full length of the root distally to involve the apex (**43A**). There are small periapical radiolucencies over the other two roots. Treatment involved root filling the mesiobuccal and palatal roots and resection of the distobuccal root. A silver point was used for obturation of the mesiobuccal root canal, because of its narrow and extremely curved nature. Gutta percha was used to obturate the palatal canal, and the distobuccal root amputation site was sealed with amalgam. Finally, the occlusal access cavity was restored with amalgam. As a result of this treatment the inflammatory lesion resolved with normal bony healing.

44 (a) There is a well-defined ovoid radiolucency enveloping the crown of the unerupted $\overline{6|}$. The lesion has displaced the $\overline{6|}$ inferiorly, the developing $\overline{7|}$ distally, and caused almost complete resorption of the distal root $\overline{E|}$.

(b) Dentigerous cyst – these cysts arise from the reduced enamel epithelium which surrounds the crown of an unerupted tooth. They are more common before middle age, and are most often found in relation to unerupted lower third molars and maxillary canines. Typically, they appear as well-defined, often corticated radiolucencies, usually positioned symmetrically around the crown of an unerupted tooth, although in some cases the cyst may be located to one side of the crown. The width of a normal follicular space around the crown of an unerupted tooth is usually 2–3 mm; if it is greater than this, a cyst or tumour should be suspected. Superimposition of a radiolucent lesion upon the crown of an unerupted tooth may appear to resemble a dentigerous cyst, but in the example illustrated, the crown lies within the lesion.

(c) The management of this example would involve marsupialization of the cyst and the exposure of $\overline{6|}$ to allow its eruption, as it still has eruptive potential (indicated by incompletely formed roots). The excised portion of cyst lining should be sent for histological examination to confirm the provisional diagnosis. The cyst cavity may require packing to prevent early closure of the surgical opening and thus delay the eruption of $\overline{6|}$ In addition, $\overline{E|}$ requires extraction because of the extensive amount of resorption of its distal root.

In those situations where it is not practicable to allow the involved tooth to erupt, the cyst should be enucleated and the associated tooth removed.

45   1, Ear lobe; 2, soft palate; 3, right inferior turbinate; 4, hard palate; 5, double image of hard palate from the right hand side; 6, dorsum of the tongue; 7, body of the hyoid bone.

46   No, there is no need to alter normal radiographic selection criteria because the patient is pregnant. The risk of genetic abnormalities is infinitesimal (5×10^{-7} using rectangular collimation and E-speed film at 70 kV with 20 cm focus to skin distance) compared with their natural frequency at birth of $1–3 \times 10^{-2}$. Similar considerations apply to the risk of cancer induction.

47   Yes, both of the restorations are inappropriately contoured, having no contact point between $|67$ and overhanging interproximal cervical margins, resulting in stagnation areas for plaque retention. There is bone loss of the alveolar crest immediately below the overhanging amalgam restorations, due to localized chronic periodontitis.

48 (a) Severe hypodontia, the only permanent teeth present being $1|1$ and $\overline{632|236}$. Hypodontia usually affects only the permanent dentition. In less severe forms of hypodontia the teeth most commonly missing are upper lateral incisors, lower second premolars, and upper and lower third molars. Even in severe forms it is unusual for the first molars and upper central incisors to be missing.

(b) Ectodermal dysplasia, a congenital ectodermal defect characterized by hypohidrosis, hypotrichosis, and hypodontia. It is usually of x-linked inheritance, but it has been reported in women with autosomal recessive inheritance. The young child often presents with a 'fever of unknown origin' in the first year of life because of disordered temperature regulation associated with a partial or complete absence of sweat glands. The skin is dry and sometimes feels scaly, due to a reduction in the number of sebaceous glands. The hair, particularly that of the scalp and eyebrows, is fine, scanty, and often blonde. The facial features are characteristic, with frontal bossing, a depressed nasal bridge, and a reduced lower face height.

The oral manifestations are variable; the hypodontia is usually associated with a reduction in tooth size, with the upper central incisors often being conical in shape. This is not the situation illustrated in the question. The alveolus fails to develop in the regions where teeth are absent, so causing a reduction of vertical dimension and protuberance of the lips. Treatment in those severely affected normally consists of a combination of orthodontic and advanced restorative techniques.

49 (a) There is a ragged patchy destruction of the body of the mandible on both sides – the so-called moth-eaten appearance. A poorly defined radiolucency extends from the alveolar crest throughout the full thickness of the body of the mandible and involves the lower border, and on the left side it appears that a pathological fracture has occurred.

(b) Osteoradionecrosis – the high doses of radiation used in radiotherapy cause endarteritis obliterans, which greatly reduces the blood supply and the reparative powers of bone, particularly in the mandible. Subsequent trauma (e.g., tooth extraction, as in this case) usually leads to infection and osteoradionecrosis, with sequestra formation and discharging sinuses. A knowledge of the previous radiotherapy is important in reaching a diagnosis.

(c) (i) Osteomyelitis.

(ii) Primary malignant and metastatic tumours of bone.

The history, signs, and symptoms usually aid the diagnosis.

50 (a) There is enlargement of the mandible with a skeletal class III jaw relationship. The supra-orbital ridges are more prominent than normal and the frontal sinuses are enlarged. The pituitary fossa is of normal shape, but its dimensions are greater than normal, however there is thinning of the bony outline of the posterior margin of the pituitary fossa.

(b) Acromegaly.

(c) Acromegaly arises from secretion of growth hormone from the cells of the anterior pituitary gland after general body growth has ceased. This is most commonly due to formation of an adenoma of the anterior lobe of the pituitary gland. The growth of this tumour produces enlargement and often destruction of the outline of the pituitary fossa.

(d) Most bones after puberty are incapable of continued growth due to the fusion of the epiphyses. However, some bones (such as the mandible and the bones of the hands), have articular surfaces which, when stimulated by excess growth hormone production, have the potential for further growth. In addition, the excess growth hormone secretion results in hypertrophy of some of the soft tissues, such as the lips and tongue. Thus, clinical features include:

(i) Lengthening of the ascending ramus and body of the mandible.
(ii) Enlargement of the hands and feet.
(iii) Coarsening of the facial features.
(iv) Enlargement of the tongue, causing buccal inclination of the teeth.
If the abnormal secretion of the growth hormone occurs before closure of the epiphyseal plates, there is a generalized enlargement of the bones so that the patient becomes much taller than normal (gigantism).

51 **1**, Lateral wall of the floor of the nose; **2**, outline of the maxillary antrum; **3**, incisive canal; **4**, root of zygoma.

52 (a) Removal of a silver-point root filling from the upper right central incisor with a trepan.
(b) The radiograph has been taken to help determine the relationship of the trepan to the silver point. It shows that the trepan has not been directed in the long axis of the silver point, but inclined mesially, and that the cutting edges at the end of the trepan are flared. The problems that might arise from this situation are excess removal of radicular dentine or fracture of the instrument.

53 (a) Elongation of the images of upper molars in periapical films may arise from either one of two errors in technique – insufficient downwards beam angulation or bending of the film in the vault of the palate. Investigate the problem by examining a sample of films. Bending errors can be distinguished by the greater degree of elongation of the apical regions of the tooth roots than of the coronal aspects. This,and insufficient beam angle, can lead to the apices not being recorded on the radiograph, although this fault can also arise from incorrect film position.
Solve the problem by introducing film holders and the paralleling technique. Holders prevent film bending and the paralleling technique avoids the need to determine the amount of downwards angle. In the interim advise Mr A to increase his beam angle and to instruct his patients not to press the film too hard into the palate.
(b) Generally, totally black films can be due to complete exposure to light or to X-rays, or to overdevelopment of the film. Light fogging to this degree could be a result of opening the film packet inadvertently in unsafe light conditions. X-ray fogging could be caused by an intermittently faulty exposure timer on the X-ray set, a possibility that should be investigated urgently. Overdevelopment could be due to hot or overconcentrated developer solution (developer often comes as a concentrate) or to leaving the film too long in the developer solution.
As this is an intermittent problem limited to Ms B, it is unlikely that the developer temperature or concentration is responsible. Ask staff who carry out the processing of the films if they have any memory of accidentally opening the film packet in daylight or of leaving the radiograph in the developer solution for too long. Ensure that this inquiry is done in a nonthreatening, 'off the record' way, as you may not get an honest answer! Most importantly, ensure, as soon as possible, that the X-

ray machine in Ms B's surgery is checked by a qualified X-ray engineer.

54 (a) The image has been formed by reformatting the data obtained from the original series of axial (horizontal) scans, into a vertical slice in the plane shown by the white line in the lower part of the illustration. Reformatted images are less clear than those obtained by direct scanning, but it is difficult to obtain direct computerized tomographic scans in the sagittal plane, which are necessary for implant assessment.

(b) A periapical radiograph is also required to assess the bone quality at the intended site of the implant and the condition of adjacent teeth and bone.

55 There is silver-point root filling which:

(i) Projects well beyond the apex of the tooth.

(ii) Has perforated the root on its buccal aspect, as determined from the parallax views. **55A** is centred on ⌐12 and the post appears to lie within the root canal. In **55B**, the tube has moved distally to be centred on ⌐23, but the root filling now appears to be more mesially placed relative to the root canal ⌐2. In effect, the image of the root filling has moved in the opposite direction to that taken by the X-ray tube, thus indicating that the root filling lies buccal to the root canal.

In **55A**, the periodontal ligament space just below its mid portion is widened on both sides of the root, suggesting there is a localized inflammatory response at the site of the perforation.

56 (a) **1**, Oblique ridge; **2**, mylohyoid ridge; **3**, inferior alveolar canal.

(b) The mandible is narrower in this part of the jaw as there is a concavity, below the mylohyoid ridge, which accommodates the contents of the submandibular space, e.g., the submandibular salivary gland and lymph node. Above the mylohyoid ridge the bone is more dense, because it is broader (to contain the tooth roots); it also contains more bony trabeculae resulting from the functional stresses transmitted to the bone by the tooth roots.

57 An exostosis or cancellous osteoma, both of which may occur as outgrowths of new bone with radiologically normal internal architecture; they are mostly indistinguishable radiographically. Exostoses are hyperplasias with limited growth potential that are genetically and/or functionally determined, whereas osteomas are benign neoplasms. Both are slow-growing. The most common exostoses in the jaws are the palatal and mandibular tori. An osteoma may be either cancellous or compact in composition, the latter appearing as a uniformly radiopaque, circumscribed mass. Both may arise either centrally or peripherally in the jaws. Osteomas, rarely, may be multiple, in which case a diagnosis of Gardner's syndrome should be considered. In addition to the bone tumours, patients with this syndrome may have intestinal polyposis (which are prone to undergo malignant transformation), supernumerary teeth, sebaceous cysts, and fibromas in the skin.

58 (a) The patient is edentulous, apart from a retained unerupted lower right third molar. There is an elongated multilocular radiolucent lesion involving the right angle of the mandible and most of the ascending ramus up to the sigmoid notch. It is well-defined and partly corticated, with loss of the bony outline of the anterior aspect of the ascending ramus. The alveolar canal and its contents are displaced inferiorly and posteriorly. The crown of the tooth is probably carious, but there is no resorption of the root.

(b) A postero-anterior (rotated) radiograph, requested to assess the extent of the buccal or lingual bony expansion of the mandible and the condition of the remaining bone. There is slight expansion, with some thinning of both buccal and lingual cortical plates. The loculated nature of the lesion, the inferior alveolar canal, and the carious lesion in the molar tooth are all clearly visible.

(c) The differential diagnosis of a loculated lesion in this part of the jaw includes an odontogenic keratocyst (as in this example) or an ameloblastoma. A dentigerous cyst is possible, but less likely, in view of the elongated, loculated appearance and age of the patient (dentigerous cysts occur more commonly in younger patients).

(d) Follow-up radiographs are particularly indicated for odontogenic keratocysts, which have a 10–20% incidence of recurrence. Radiographic review should continue for a minimum of 5 years, during which period the majority of recurrences occur.

59   **59A** shows a short, closed pointer cone from a set which operates at 50 kV. With the X-ray tube placed at the front of the tube housing, the focal spot to skin distance is short (10 cm) so that the emergent X-ray beam is divergent, making it unsuitable for the paralleling technique. In addition, the plastic material of the pointer causes some of the emergent X-ray beam to scatter, increasing patient and operator exposure. In contrast, the dental set in **59B** operates at 60–70 kV and has a continuous, lead-lined, round, open-ended spacer cone. Here, the focal spot is situated at the rear of the tube head (arrow), resulting in a long (30 cm) focal spot to cone end distance. Consequently, the emergent X-ray beam is far less divergent than that from the spacer cone in **59A**, and is therefore suitable for the paralleling technique. The open end of the cone minimizes scatter of the emergent X-ray beam.

In the United Kingdom there are statutory requirements for the focal spot to skin distance. For sets operating at 60 kV and less, the minimum distance is 10 cm, and for sets operating above 60 kV, the minimum distance is 20 cm.

60 (a) Extensive alveolar bone loss is present around the newly erupted lower incisor teeth. These changes suggest a diagnosis of prepubertal periodontitis. The tooth apices are incompletely formed, as would be expected at this age.

(b) Prepubertal periodontitis is usually associated with some form of systemic disease, which predisposes the periodontal tissues to rapid bone destruction. Such systemic conditions include:
(i) Langerhan's cell histiocytosis (histiocytosis X), as in this patient.
(ii) Juvenile onset diabetes
(iii) Adrenocortical hyperfunction (Cushing's syndrome).
(iv) Papillon–Lefevre syndrome.
(v) Hypophosphatasia.
(vi) Chediak–Higashi syndrome.

61   **1**, Pterygoid plate; **2**, pterygoid hamulus; **3**, maxillary tuberosity; **4**, root of the zygoma.

62 (a) There is an oblique fracture of the left angle of the mandible running through the distal aspect of the socket of the third molar. This is a horizontally unfavourable fracture and the distal fragment has been pulled upwards by the masseter and temporalis muscles. The malalignment is particularly clear at the lower border of the mandible and at the cortical margins of the inferior alveolar canal.

(b) The postero-anterior radiograph shows the medial displacement of the posterior fragment of the mandible. It also displays the condyles well. One of the elements in determining the treatment modality for many fractures is the degree and direction of displacement of the fragments.

(c) Fracture of the neck of the opposite condyle. In fractures of one side of the mandible, particularly caused by a direct blow, a 'contra-coup' fracture of the opposite condylar neck may occur, as a result of transmitted force.

(d) Assuming that there are no other serious injuries, the fracture should be reduced and the fragments fixed under a general anaesthetic. In addition, consideration should be given to the removal of $\overline{8|}$, which lies in the fracture site. Controversy exists regarding the management of a tooth in the line of the fracture, so a conservative approach is often adopted. In general, however, a tooth should be extracted if:
(i) It interferes with the reduction of the fracture.
(ii) The tooth is fractured, particularly if the root is involved, or the tooth vitality is compromised.
(iii) The tooth is extensively decayed or is associated with disease, such as periapical inflammation.
In addition, the presence of a tooth in the fracture line may imply a compound fracture (i.e.,the fracture communicates with the oral cavity via the periodontal ligament).
Thus, the management of this case may involve:
(i) The prescription of a course of an appropriate antibiotic, and analgesics as required.
(ii) Removal (if necessary) of $\overline{8|}$ using a surgical approach.
(iii) Reduction of the fracture, using temporary intermaxillary fixation to obtain the correct occlusal relationship.
(iv) Rigid internal fixation using a bone plate (e.g., miniplate).
(v) Immediate post-operative radiographs to assess the treatment of the fracture (e.g., dental panoramic tomograph, postero-anterior radiograph).
(vi) Post-operative advice on diet and oral hygiene, and instigation of follow-up care.

63 (a) The crown has two amalgam restorations. There is an elongated pulp chamber and a larger than normal distance from the enamel–cement junction to the root bifurcation; consequently, the tooth has two relatively short roots.

(b) Taurodontism, which can affect any tooth, but is most often seen in the mandibular molar or premolar teeth. It may occur singly or involve several teeth.

64 (a) The bridge has become loose at 2|, because the core of the jacket crown preparation has fractured, as illustrated by the horizontal radiolucent fracture line at gingival level.

(b) The bridge could be sectioned from 2|, converting it to a cantilever design. Endodontic treatment could then be completed for 2|and a post crown provided.

(c) Remnants of platinum foil left behind on the fitting surface of the porcelain jacket crown.

65 (a) A multilocular radiolucency is present in the body of the mandible, extending from the mesial root of the lower left first molar to the unerupted third molar and from the upper border of the alveolus towards the lower border. It has a smooth, well-defined margin, which is scalloped and of variable cortication. There is resorption of the roots of the lower first molar and the alveolar crest has been expanded superiorly between the molar teeth. There is no evidence of calcification within the lesion other than the radiopaque septa which create the multilocular appearance.

(b) Other useful radiographic views would include:

(i) A dental panoramic tomograph to show the full extent of the lesion and the remainder of the mandible, including the contralateral side, or right and left oblique lateral views of the mandible.

(ii) A lower true (90°) occlusal radiograph to assess possible buccolingual expansion in the body of the mandible.

(iii) A postero-anterior radiograph of the mandible if the lesion is shown to extend into the angle and/or ramus, to demonstrate any mediolateral expansion in this area.

(c) Radiological differential diagnosis in this age group includes ameloblastoma or odontogenic myxoma as the most likely possibilities, in view of the site of the lesion, its multilocular expansive nature, and the presence of root resorption. Less likely possibilities are a giant cell lesion or odontogenic keratocyst. Histologically, the lesion was a myxoma – a non-invasive odontogenic tumour originating from fibroblasts of a tooth germ, which produce excessive ground substance. Treatment is by surgical removal and careful follow-up.

66 (a) An upper anterior (standard) occlusal radiograph.

(b) There is an ovoid, well-defined, and corticated radiolucency situated in the midline just above the apices of the upper central incisor teeth. It measures approximately 25 mm by 10 mm. The lesion has encroached upon the anterior aspect of the floor of the nose, which has been partially resorbed.

(c) Anterior nasal spine.

(d) Nasopalatine (incisive canal) cyst. These arise from epithelial remnants of the nasopalatine duct. On an intra-oral radiograph, the width of a normal incisive foramen rarely exceeds 6 mm and its outline tends not to be corticated. If it is greater than this and also corticated, an abnormality should be suspected. Nasopalatine cysts may be projected above the apices of the central incisors, as in this example, or between the roots of the central incisors, when differentiation from an apical inflammatory lesion may be more difficult. These cysts originate in the midline, but occasionally eccentric growth may produce an asymmetric radiolucency. Long-standing cysts may reach a considerable size and cause thinning and expansion of the bony cortical plates.

(e) In most cases, the cyst should be enucleated, usually from the palatal aspect. Recurrence is uncommon.

67 (i) Periapical inflammation associated with $\overline{6|}$. The lower right first molar is heavily restored and root filled. There is an ovoid radiolucency around the apex of the mesial root $\overline{6|}$, typical of a periapical inflammatory lesion. In addition, there is widening apically of the periodontal ligament space of the distal root and a small radiopaque body, probably endodontic filling material, close to the distal root surface just above the apex.

(ii) Osteoarthrosis of the right TMJ. There is flattening of the condylar head with anterior lipping. This appearance is seen in degenerative joint disease, and the marked attrition of the occlusal surfaces of the teeth indicate heavy functional wear. However, osteoarthrosis of the TMJ does not always cause discomfort, particularly in the older patient. The radiographic appearance of a well-defined flattened surface with the absence of erosion or sclerosis suggests that the condition may be inactive and represents past disease.

(iii) There are large restorations present in most of the teeth, so pulpitis associated with any one of these is a possible source of the patient's discomfort.

68 **1**, Root of the zygoma; **2**, zygomatic arch; **3**, floor of the antrum.

69 (a) Strip perforation of the root in the furcal region, which has resulted from misdirected instrumentation during the preparation of the root canal. The risk of this occurrence may be reduced by using the anticurvature filing technique and by avoiding excessively large Gates Glidden burs during preparation of the canal.

(b) Small strip perforations may be treated conservatively, but larger ones may require a surgical approach. In this example, the mesial root and the mesial half of the crown of the tooth were resected, because of the position of the perforation and the associated bone loss in the furcal region.

70 (a) There is a gross caries of $\overline{87|}$ and $\underline{5|}$ with diffuse periapical radiolucent areas $\overline{87|}$ In addition, $\dfrac{3|\ 3\ \ 5}{4|\ \ 45}$ are unerupted and, with the exception of 5, are deeply placed.

There is a complex odontome $\overline{4|}$ region, a supernumerary tooth or fragment of root $\underline{|3}$ and $\overline{|D}$ is retained. On the left side there is a well-defined radiopaque mass in the mandibular ramus and at the lower border of the mandible, both of which have an appearance consistent with an osteoma or an exostosis. Similarly, the small rounded radiopacity overlying the left maxillary antrum and root of the zygoma is probably an osteoma. The alveolar bone of the maxilla and mandibular body show widespread patchy radiopacities, the appearance of which is characteristic of multiple enostoses or osteomas.

(b) An acute exacerbation of chronic periapical inflammation $\overline{87}$

(c) Familial adenomatous polyposis (Gardner's syndrome). This is an inherited condition with an autosomal dominant pattern. It is characterized by the formation of multiple osteomas, which are most frequently found in the skull, particularly the frontal bones and facial bones. The syndrome is also associated with the presence of unerupted teeth and odontome formation. Other features include skin lesions such as sebaceous cysts, subcutaneous fibromas and lipomas, and are frequently followed (usually before middle age) by the formation of multiple adenomatous polyps of the large intestine. The polyps carry a high risk of developing into adenocarcinomas.

(d) Proctosigmoidoscopy and a barium enema and/or meal to ascertain whether intestinal polyps are present. Biopsy of the polyps, when present, to allow appropriate management of these premalignant or malignant lesions.

71 (a) There is a large amalgam restoration, which is retained by distal and mesial pins. The mesial one has been incorrectly angled in relation to the long axis of the tooth and has perforated the mesial aspect of the crown $\overline{7}$ and penetrated the adjacent alveolar bone.

(b) The loss of $\overline{6}$ has permitted $\overline{7}$ to tilt mesially. There is, however, very little of the coronal tissue left to indicate the actual orientation of the long axis of $\overline{7}$, and placement of a pin vertically into the root dentine has resulted in perforation.

(c) Perforation of the crown could have been avoided by taking a preoperative bitewing or periapical radiograph and by assessing the root angulation clinically using a periodontal probe.

(d) As the pin has penetrated the tooth surface, its removal is indicated since it is likely to become a focus for inflammation. However, retrieval from an orthograde direction might be difficult because, in removing the investing amalgam restoration, the coronal part of the pin may also be destroyed. Thus, there may be insufficient material of the pin left to grasp and unscrew. Alternatively, a surgical procedure, involving both buccal and lingual flap reflection to visualize the pin, would allow it to be sectioned at the root surface and the remaining portion to be removed from the bone. A restoration should be placed to seal the perforation in the tooth.

72 (a) The primary canine and first and second primary molars have erupted into the mouth. A pulpotomy has been carried out on the first primary molar with radiopaque filling material obturating the whole of the coronal pulp chamber. There is a mesial restoration in the second primary molar. The first permanent molar is unerupted, but calcification of the enamel is complete. Also unerupted, but developing, are the permanent canine and first premolar, but the second premolar is not present and there is no resorption of the roots of the second primary molar

(b) The patient is 4–5 years of age; the first permanent molar crown has completed its formation, which normally occurs at around 3 years, but it is not yet close to eruption, which is usually at 6–7 years.

(c) The second premolar tooth is absent and there is no evidence of a radiolucent tooth germ. Normally, mineralization in this tooth starts at approximately two and a half years of age, but can be much later. It is probable that in this child the tooth is congenitally absent; however, it is also possible that the tooth is ectopically placed, in which case a dental panoramic tomograph is needed to determine its position.

73 (a) There is widespread ragged destruction of the body of the mandible, much of it having the so-called moth-eaten appearance, extending through its full thickness and containing small opaque pieces of bone (sequestra). The margin of the destroyed area is poorly defined. Anteriorly, the mandible appears more radiopaque and sclerotic near the lower border, suggesting reactive bone formation has occurred although there is no evidence of new subperiosteal bone. A pathological fracture is present through the left angle.

(b) Osteomyelitis – a spreading inflammation of bone and bone marrow resulting in the destruction of the infected bone. In this case the lesion arose from the infected lower molar and became exacerbated by the patient's diabetic condition, which caused a decreased resistance to infection. The sclerosis of the surrounding bone suggests that the osteomyelitis has entered a chronic phase. Treatment would involve long-term antibiotic therapy, together with the removal of necrotic bone (sequestra) as necessary.

(c) Similar ragged moth-eaten destruction of bone is seen in:
(i) Osteoradionecrosis.
(ii) Primary or secondary malignant tumours involving bone.
The history and presenting signs and symptoms usually allow a clinical differential diagnosis (see **49** and **81**).

(d) The hyoid bone.

74 There is no mandatory requirement for the routine use of lead aprons. The *Guidance Notes* to *The Ionising Radiations Regulations* (1985) specify that, in dental radiography, a lead apron should be used during the examination of a woman who is, or who may be pregnant, if there is a possibility that the fetus would be irradiated by the primary beam. This is only likely to happen in the case of a vertex occlusal projection. With good technique (e.g. the use of rectangular collimation, E-speed film, and the paralleling technique) the radiation dose is infinitesimal. Further, even under a lead apron there is an irreducible minimum of scattered radiation that reaches the gonads through the chest and abdomen. However, a lead apron is needed to protect a parent or carer supporting a child or handicapped adult patient who is undergoing a radiographic examination.

75 **1**, Lateral wall of the floor of the nose; **2**, incisive canal; **3**, anterior wall of the maxillary antrum.

ANSWERS

76 (a) The apical portion of 5⌋ appears to lie within the right maxillary antrum. The root, which is upside-down, contains a root filling. The cortical lamina outlining the antral floor is discontinuous at the site of the 5⌋ socket, at which point there are several small dense radiopaque fragments.

(b) In view of persistent discomfort it is probable that the maxillary antrum has become infected. An occipitomental radiograph should be taken to assess whether there is mucosal thickening or a fluid level within the antrum.

(c) Infection of the maxillary antrum, if present, must be treated. Then the root should be removed, probably using a Caldwell–Luc approach, and the 5⌋ socket curetted and closed by advancing a mucoperiosteal flap.

77 (a) There is a radiolucent fracture line through the neck of the right condyle and the condylar fragment is displaced posteriorly. The bone of the condylar process is radiolucent and ill-defined, and there is some irregularity of the outline of the sigmoid notch.

(b) A malignant tumour involving the mandibular condyle and resulting in a pathological fracture. The history is suggestive of temporomandibular joint dysfunction, but the fracture of the condylar neck and the ill-defined radiolucency of the condylar region indicate the presence of a destructive lesion.

(c) Although primary malignant tumours occasionally arise in this part of the mandible, a metastatic deposit from a primary tumour elsewhere in the body is the more likely diagnosis. The most common primary tumours with jaw metastases arise from the breast, bronchus, thyroid, kidney, and prostate. It would be necessary, therefore, to investigate the local lesion further to determine its extent and nature, and, where appropriate, to examine the rest of the body for a possible primary tumour.

Further investigation of the condylar lesion might include a postero-anterior radiograph of the condyles, computerized tomography (**77A**) or MRI to determine whether there is spread of the tumour into the adjacent soft tissues and/or dependent lymph nodes. A bone scintiscan (**77B**) will help to confirm the presence and extent of the destructive lesion, and a skeletal bone scintiscan may be undertaken if other skeletal metastases are suspected.

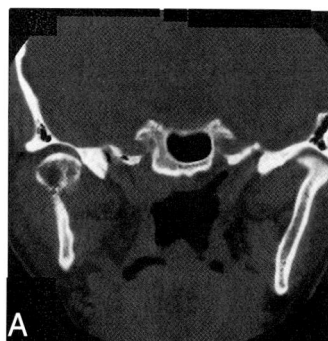
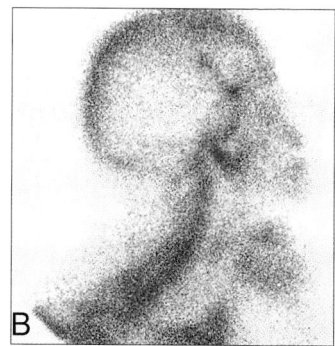

Biopsy is indicated to determine the histological nature of the lesion. To evaluate the site of the primary tumour, further appropriate clinical examination and radiological, biochemical, haematological, and histological tests are necessary.

78 (a) This patient is approximately 14–15 years' old, as determined by the state of root development of the teeth, and is undergoing fixed appliance orthodontic treatment.

(b) Both upper second premolars are unerupted, but the image of 5| is magnified and ill-defined, as it lies palatally to the dental arch and so is not fully within the focal trough of the tomograph. There is an enlarged follicular space around the crown of 5, indicating cystic change. All the third molars are unerupted and at an early stage of formation. The upper ones appear to be developing normally; however, the lower ones are orientated transversely.

(c) The unerupted upper premolars may interfere with the orthodontic movement of adjacent teeth and thus delay the achievement of a satisfactory alignment of the dentition. It is now accepted by most clinicians that unerupted lower third molars do not contribute to lower incisor crowding.

(d) There is an irregularly rounded area of radiopacity, approximately 1 cm in diameter, below the apex of the lower right canine surrounded by normal bone. This appearance is typical of a localized area of osteosclerosis and does not require any treatment. Osteosclerosis probably occurs in response to chronic low-grade irritation, the cause of which is not always obvious as it may have been associated with the primary dentition. It is most commonly seen in the lower premolar/molar region of the mandible.

79 (a) The radiolucency represents part of the maxillary antrum. The appearance is due to a loculus separated from the main part of the antrum by an unusually thick septal wall. The appearance may be misinterpreted as an abnormality, such as a cyst or benign neoplasm. The presence of vascular channels within the radiolucency, a normal anatomical feature, indicates that it is part of the maxillary antrum. In cases where doubt persists, further radiographs may be required for comparison with the opposite side, allowing a more complete antral examination.

(b) (i) There is some foreshortening of the teeth due to the vertical angulation of the X-ray tube being too great.
(ii) The bottom right-hand corner of the radiograph has not been exposed due to incorrect centring of the tube relative to the film (coning).

80 1, Nasal fossa; **2**, lateral wall of the floor of the nose; **3**, incisive foramen; **4**, median suture; **5**, outline of the tip of the nose.

81 (a) There is a poorly defined, ragged radiolucent area of bone destruction in the middle of the left ascending ramus – the so-called moth-eaten appearance. The buccal cortical plate in the region of the angle has been destroyed and perforated.

(b) A malignant neoplasm – the radiographic appearance indicates a destructive lesion, but does not allow the distinction between a primary or secondary tumour to be made. However, metastatic lesions are more common in the jaws than are primary malignant tumours, and this example turned out to be a metastasis. Metastases in the jaws most commonly arise from primary tumours in the bronchus, breast, kidney, thyroid and prostate, and typically occur where residues of haematopoietic marrow may persist.

(c) (i) A dental panoramic tomograph or an oblique lateral radiograph of the left angle and ramus of the mandible, as they would provide a view of the lesion at right angles to that of the original radiograph.

(ii) A computerized tomographic scan to assess the size and possible spread of the lesion into the surrounding soft tissues and dependent lymph nodes.

(d) Radioisotope bone scanning, using a bone-seeking isotope.

(e) A similar ragged moth-eaten appearance is also seen in:

(i) Osteoradionecrosis.

(ii) Osteomyelitis.

The history and presenting signs and symptoms usually allow a clinical differential diagnosis (**49** and **73**).

82 (a) There is a radiopacity, which has a horizontal menisciform upper margin (typical of a fluid level) in the lower aspect of the left maxillary antrum. There is also a slightly lobulated radiopaque shadow at the roof of the antrum, suggestive of thickened antral lining. The contralateral maxillary antrum seems normal. The overall appearance is that of a unilateral maxillary sinusitis.

(b) The failure of the socket to heal, together with the development of the sinus infection, suggests the presence of an oro-antral fistula. When the fistula is large, fluid from the mouth passes into the antrum and thence to the nasal airway, to be swallowed or passed via the nostrils. If the fistulous tract is narrow, there is poor drainage between the mouth and the antrum, which predisposes to the development of sinusitis, as in this example.

(c) The management consists of:

(i) Resolution of the infection by drainage of the maxillary antrum and antibiotic therapy.

(ii) Followed by closure of the oro-antral fistula by an advancement flap procedure.

83 (a) There is a well-delineated, dome-shaped, uniformly radiopaque mass occupying the lower half of the maxillary antrum. It does not appear to have expanded or resorbed the bony outline of the antral floor, which remains intact. (Note that it is important to compare the appearance of the abnormal side with that of the opposite side. In this example, the right maxillary antrum is normal, although the antral floor has extended inferiorly into alveolar bone previously occupied by 6⌋, resulting in a somewhat loculated appearance.)

(b) Antral mucosal cyst – these are thought to arise following obstruction of the duct of a seromucous gland, or within a thickened antral lining or mucosal polyp of a chronically inflamed antrum. They occur most often in young adults and are usually asymptomatic, being discovered as an incidental radiographic finding. Antral mucosal cysts are of variable size, occasionally bilateral, and most commonly are found on the antral floor, which they do not resorb. Because they develop within the antral cavity and not the bone, they do not have a bony cortical outline, which helps to distinguish them from odontogenic cysts. Typically, there is no expansion of the maxillary antrum.

(c) Antral polyp, odontogenic or post-operative maxillary cyst enlarging into the antral cavity, and an antral neoplasm. It is not always possible to differentiate on a dental panoramic tomograph between mucosal cysts and antral polyps, although the latter are usually associated with a more generalized thickening of the antral lining. Odontogenic cysts expand from the alveolus into the antral cavity, and so are usually separated from the residual antral cavity by a thin lamina of bone. Antral neoplasms are usually malignant and show destruction of part of the bone of the antral wall.

(d) No treatment is required because antral mucosal cysts usually resolve spontaneously. In those instances when chronic periapical disease is thought to have produced inflammatory changes within the antral lining, appropriate treatment of the relevant tooth is indicated. If there is doubt about the nature of the lesion, further investigation is necessary.

84 (a) Upper anterior (standard) occlusal (**84A**) and periapical (**84B**) radiographs of the left upper central incisor region.

(b) There is a tuberculate and mesiodens supernumerary teeth overlying the palatal (as determined by vertical parallax) aspect of the crown of the left upper incisor, so preventing it from erupting. For the occlusal radiograph, there is a steeper inclination of the X-ray tube to the vertical plane than for the periapical radiograph. Thus, the X-ray tube has swung downwards from a more vertical angulation to a more horizontal one. Similarly, the supernumerary teeth (being palatally placed), have moved in the same direction as that taken by the tube, relative to the unerupted central incisor.

(c) Surgical removal of the supernumerary tooth and exposure of the central incisor with bonding of an orthodontic bracket, so that the unerupted central incisor can be actively extruded using an orthodontic appliance. Traction is necessary because the root of the central incisor is already well-developed and thus its natural eruptive potential is low.

85 (a) The top part of the film is largely unexposed and distorted, because it was bent or folded in the palate to such a degree that the image of the lead backing has appeared. In addition, there is overlap of the contact points of the teeth, because the horizontal beam angulation was oblique to the film.

(b) The unexposed, distorted area on the film could have been avoided by placing the longer axis horizontally (which is the conventional way for posterior teeth) rather than vertically, and by instructing the patient not to use excessive finger pressure. The overlap of the contact points could have been prevented by ensuring that the X-ray beam was at right angles to the film in the horizontal plane. Both problems might have been avoided by using a film holder with a suitable beam-aiming device.

ANSWERS

86 (a) The root canal contains an inadequately condensed filling, which is short of the apex, where the periodontal ligament space is widened. There is a well-defined, ovoid radiolucency close to the alveolar crest, which is partly superimposed upon the mesial aspect of the root. Widening of the apical periodontal ligament space suggests inadequate instrumentation and sealing of the root canal. The lesion producing the mesial radiolucency has arisen from a lateral perforation of the root during access cavity preparation.

(b) The coronal restoration should be removed, together with the existing root filling, and the root canal reinstrumented and refilled. It may be possible to seal the lateral perforation at the same time by an internal approach, provided it is small. Follow-up radiographs are necessary to determine whether the radiolucency has resolved. If a conservative approach is not possible, the perforation may be sealed with a suitable restoration, after raising a mucoperiosteal flap. At the same time, the soft tissue occupying the area of bone loss can be curetted and sent for histological examination. Such a radiolucency may be caused by an inflammatory lesion, such as a granuloma or radicular cyst. More rarely, it may be caused by other forms of odontogenic cyst or tumour.

87 (a) Following crown preparation and cementation there has been tertiary dentine formation, leading to recession of the coronal part of the pulp chamber, making a straight line access for root canal instrumentation difficult. In addition, the tooth has two fine narrow root canals in the apical two-thirds of the root, which are probably buccally and palatally positioned. The abrupt narrowing of the root canal space in the mid-root region is an important indicator of a likely bifurcation of the root canal.

(b) To obtain adequate access to the root canal, the cavity would need to be close to, or possibly through, the incisal edge of the crown. The exact position of the two root canals could be established from parallax diagnostic working length radiographs.

88 (a) No, because the radiograph is a two-dimensional representation of a three-dimensional situation. The diagnosis could be made clinically by horizontal probing (bone sounding), performed with a sharp probe under local analgesia.

(b) The defect was caused by plaque retention leading to localized chronic periodontitis. The plaque retention was promoted by a combination of poor bridge design and an abnormal curvature of the distal aspect of the root, although the latter is not clearly shown.

(c) The tooth is a bridge abutment, so it is important to try to obtain improved bony support. As the defect is three-walled, guided tissue regeneration with a permeable membrane is the treatment of choice. **88B** shows the same area 15 months after surgery. The speckled radiopacities beneath the pontic are particles of amalgam, most likely introduced into the tissues at the time of the extraction of the missing teeth.

89 (a) (i) A dental panoramic tomograph to show the full extent of the lesion and for comparison with the other side of the jaw.
(ii) A lower true (90°) occlusal radiograph centred on the left side to assess possible buccolingual bone expansion.

(b) The radiolucency is unilocular, but with a scalloped margin (hence the differing degrees of radiodensity), the upper aspect of which arches up between the roots of the molar teeth. It has a smooth, but undulating outline, which is moderately well-defined but not corticated. It does not appear to have displaced or resorbed the teeth.

(c) The features described, particularly the scalloped outline around the roots of the teeth, suggest a diagnosis of solitary bone cyst. These so-called cysts are in fact air-filled cavities within the bone and they do not have an epithelial lining. The aetiology is unknown, but may be associated with previous trauma. Management is usually conservative. In some instances the lesion may regress spontaneously. More often it is necessary to expose and curette the bony wall of the cavity, following which the lesion heals.

90 The table illustrates primarily the effect of added filtration on patient entrance dose (skin dose). The X-ray beam generated by a dental X-ray set is polychromatic, containing a relative preponderance of low energy photons which are of no diagnostic value but contribute to the patient's skin dose. Beam filtration reduces this unnecessary radiation and at the same time increases the relative proportion of higher energy and diagnostically useful photons (referred to as beam hardening). This is achieved in two ways: first, there is a degree of inherent filtration in the dental X-ray tube assembly; second, by adding filtration in the form of a high atomic number metal, for instance, aluminium. The *Guidance Notes* to *The Ionising Radiations Regulations* (1985) specify a total filtration equivalent to at least 1.5 mm of aluminium for X-ray tube voltages up to and including 70 kV, and 2.5 mm above 70 kV. An additional effect of increased filtration is a prolonging of the exposure time because of the reduction in total photon fluence.

91 (a) A magnetic resonance image taken in the axial plane through the body of the mandible.

(b) There is an irregularly shaped high signal area (white) involving the floor of the mouth and the right lateral margin of the tongue, the posterior body of the mandible, and the adjacent buccal soft tissues. The low signal of the cortical plates of the mandible (appear as black) is discontinuous lingually, indicating bone destruction.
Magnetic resonance images demonstrate good soft tissue contrast and so are particularly helpful in demonstrating lesions of the soft tissues.

(c) A bone scintiscan of the head and neck.

(d) There is an area of increased uptake (hot-spot) of radionuclide in the right body of the mandible. This area appears to be larger than the area of bone destruction illustrated in the radiograph **91A**. The radiograph shows only where the mineralized bone matrix has been destroyed, but not the full extent of the tumour infiltrating through the marrow spaces.

  (e) Squamous cell carcinoma of the right floor of mouth mucosa, with local spread into the adjacent bone of the mandible.

92   (i) An antral mucosal cyst, the dome-shaped radiopacity on the floor of the maxillary antrum, overlying the roots of the molar teeth.
(ii) Sclerosing osteitis at the apex of the heavily restored lower first molar tooth.
(iii) Tonsilloliths, focal collections of dystrophic mineralization or concretions that result from previous episodes of chronic tonsillitis. In the example illustrated there are at least four radiopacities overlying the mid portion of the mandibular ramus. The lower two, just below the mandibular foramen, are clearly defined and irregularly shaped. The upper two, at the level of the mandibular foramen, are much more elongated and more diffuse in outline. These latter represent ghost (secondary) images of tonsilliths which are present on the opposite side. Tonsilloliths, radiographically, may resemble parotid gland calculi; however, the former lie lingual to, and the latter buccal to, the mandibular ramus.

93 (a) A parotid gland sialogram – sialography is the injection of a radiopaque contrast medium via the duct orifice into the ductal system of a salivary gland to demonstrate the primary and secondary ducts, so that they can be imaged by plain films, fluoroscopy, or computerized tomography.
  (b) Sialography is primarily indicated for:
(i) Obstructive conditions of the ductal system [e.g., by a sialolith (stone), stricture], when plain radiographs have failed to demonstrate the obstruction.
(ii) Chronic inflammatory disorders.
(iii) Recurrent salivary gland swelling.
Sialography is contraindicated in the presence of acute inflammation of the salivary gland and in patients with iodine hypersensitivity.
  (c) There are numerous punctate or globular collections of radiopaque contrast medium (sialectasis) distributed throughout the parotid gland. The main duct is clearly demonstrated, but the secondary ducts appear fewer than normal. This appearance occurs in chronic inflammatory disorders of the salivary gland, such as chronic parotitis (the diagnosis in this example) or Sjögren's syndrome. Further investigations, including serum immunology and labial gland biopsy, may be necessary to differentiate these two conditions (see **31**).

94 (a) There is an irregularly shaped radiopaque object in the upper right quadrant, close to the floor of the maxillary antrum. Both premolars and the first molar are missing. The bony contour of the alveolus appears to be intact. The antral cavity appears normally radiolucent, but the floor dips down into the edentulous region, and is discontinuous in the first molar region.
  (b) The appearance is that of a foreign body, but it is not dense enough to be

metallic. It is a mineralized structure, either part of a tooth displaced into the antrum or a dystrophic mineralization, such as an antrolith. A history of complications at the time of previous dental extractions might suggest the former, whereas that of recurrent upper respiratory tract infections might suggest the latter.

(c) If this is a retained portion of tooth, it is necessary to determine its exact position, which may be within the oral soft tissues, under the antral lining, or in the antral cavity. Thus, periapical radiographs and maxillary sinus radiographs are required. For the latter, the initial view would be an occipitomental radiograph, from which an assessment may be made to determine the need for further projections.

95 (a) The coronal aspect of the root is carious and at the root apex there is a bilobed radiolucency extending partly along the distal aspect of the root. The lesion, which has a maximum diameter of approximately 7 mm, is well-defined and mostly surrounded by a cortical lamina of bone. There is loss of lamina dura apically and the mass has raised and probably thinned the floor of the maxillary antrum.

(b) It is probable that the tooth root is non-vital, and therefore the differential diagnosis is that of a periapical granuloma, a periapical cyst, or a chronic periapical abscess (see **100** for comparison).

(c) The particular complications associated with the extraction of $\underline{5}$ relate to the maxillary antrum:
(i) Displacement of the root into the cavity of the maxillary antrum, which may occur because access to the root with extraction forceps may be limited, resulting in inappropriately applied force against the thinned and weakened floor of the maxillary antrum.
(ii) The creation of a communication between the mouth and the maxillary antrum (oro-antral fistula).

96 (a) There is marked hypodontia, with congenital absence of $\overline{85432|3458}$ and $\overline{854|458}$. He also has infra-occlusion of $\underline{ED|DE}$ and $\overline{ED|E}$ due to submergence of these teeth, with a bilateral open bite.

(b) The prognosis for the permanent teeth is good, but his primary teeth, except $\overline{E|E}$, have extensive root resorption. The primary molar teeth are probably ankylosed, thus creating the appearance of 'submergence' into the bone. This submergence arises because the ankylosed teeth stop erupting, but the unaffected adjacent teeth continue to do so with progressive alveolar bone development. A number of longitudinal studies indicate that ankylosed primary teeth usually exfoliate normally and should not be extracted unless a large discrepancy develops in the marginal ridge height between them and the normally erupting teeth. The prevalence of ankylosed teeth in the primary dentition is between 7 and 14%, and over 50% of patients with this condition have more than one affected tooth.

(c) His dental care should be planned on a short-, medium-, and long-term basis.

Short term:
(i) Full preventive advice, including oral hygiene instruction.
(ii) After 6 months, check clinically and radiographically whether the infra-occluded teeth have become further submerged.
Medium term:
(i) Continue preventive care.
(ii) Following the exfoliation or extraction of EDB|DE, provide a partial upper prosthesis.
(iii) Cast metal adhesive retained onlays for E|E to establish contact with the upper prosthesis.
Long term:
Consider the provision of implants and/or bridges to replace the congenitally absent teeth.

97 (a) Lateral skull (**97A**) and a postero-anterior skull (**97B**) radiographs.

(b) Multiple, round radiolucent areas in the skull vault. The lesions are well-defined, but not corticated, and are described as appearing punched out.

(c) The appearance is typical of multiple myeloma, a lymphoreticular neoplasm of bone which usually affects people over 60 years of age. It is characterized by the multifocal proliferation of plasma cells within the bone marrow, resulting in overproduction of abnormal immunoglobulins. Once in the blood stream, these immunoglobulins (consisting of abnormal heavy and light protein chains) enter the kidney filtration system. The light chains pass into the urine and are referred to as Bence-Jones protein, while the heavy chains are retained in the blood. The proliferation of the abnormal cells causes the surrounding bone to be resorbed, thus producing the multiple radiolucent lesions. The bones most commonly involved include the skull vault, as in this case, and the mandible. Other possible diagnoses include:
(i) Multiple secondary metastases.
(ii) Langerhan's cell histiocytosis (histiocytosis X); this may cause larger areas of radiolucency in the skull vault, the so-called geographic skull (see also **129**).
(iii) Gaucher's disease – this may also cause multiple speckled radiolucencies in the skull.
The latter two conditions are usually diagnosed during the first two decades of life.

98 (a) There is little or no enamel on the crowns of the teeth, which have an angular outline with wide interdental spaces and no contact points. The roots appear normal and the pulp chambers and root canals are clearly visible, except that of 1|, which is sclerosed.

(b) Amelogenesis imperfecta (hypoplastic type), a developmental disorder in which enamel formation is defective. It is a generalized condition, so that all or most of the teeth are affected in both dentitions. There are three main types – hypoplastic, hypocalcification, and hypomaturation:
(i) In the first type, there is either a generalized reduction in the thickness of enamel, so that the crowns appear smaller and more angular or squarish

than normal, or a local deficiency, so that the teeth are pitted or have annular defects.

(ii) In the hypocalcified type, the crowns are of normal size, but the enamel lacks density and is radiographically similar to that of dentine.

(iii) In the hypomaturation form, again the crowns are of normal size, but clinically appear mottled and there is poor radiographic contrast with the dentine.

(c) There has been generalized reactive dentinogenesis leading to obliteration (sclerosis) of the pulp chamber, most likely as a result of pulpal irritation over a wide area of the crown due to the lack of protective enamel.

99 (a) The upper right lateral incisor is larger than normal. It has two crowns and a single root containing two root canals. The upper right central incisor is fully formed, 2| is nearly fully formed, but 3| has only just started root formation and is unerupted.

(b) Gemination, which results when a developing tooth undergoes partial or, less frequently, complete division. In the example illustrated there has been almost complete division to produce an appearance that resembles a normal lateral incisor and an adjacent supernumerary tooth. Gemination most commonly occurs in the incisor region and may affect either dentition. The differential diagnosis includes fusion, which arises when two adjacent developing teeth combine. The result is a single tooth of larger than normal size.

100(a) An acute infection (of a previous chronic periapical inflammatory lesion).

(b) The lower right first molar has a large mesio-occlusal amalgam restoration. There is an ill-defined periapical radiolucency associated with each root apex, that on the distal root is eccentrically placed and is round, being approximately 8 mm in diameter. There is loss of the lamina dura around the apex of the distal root and the periphery of the radiolucency is continuous with the remainder of the lamina dura. The radiolucency associated with the mesial root is similar to that on the distal root, except that it is much smaller and mesially positioned relative to the tooth apex. At the periphery of both radiolucencies there is a zone of bony sclerosis (sclerosing osteitis).

(c) The differential diagnosis of a periapical radiolucency associated with a non-vital tooth is that of a periapical granuloma, a periapical cyst, or a chronic periapical abscess. When a periapical radiolucency is less than 15–20 mm in diameter it is not possible to differentiate radiographically between the three conditions, although in general cystic lesions are well-defined and more symmetrically positioned about the root apex.

101 A large artefact lies in the middle of the tomograph and corresponds in shape to two aberrant pieces of smaller (13 x 18 cm) film. The affected area is paler than the surrounding parts of the tomograph, indicating underexposure. The most probable way this could have occurred is if the aberrant films had been inside the cassette when the panoramic tomograph was exposed. The cassettes contain two intensifying screens, one on each side of the panoramic film. The aberrant pieces of film would have obstructed the fluorescence from one of the intensifying screens from reaching the panoramic film, leading to underexposure of the relevant area.

In addition, there are radiopaque artefacts of retained ear-rings (primary shadows) and their corresponding secondary ('ghost') shadows overlying the maxillary antra. Ear-rings or other detachable metallic objects should always be removed from the facial region before panoramic tomography because of the artefacts they produce. The secondary shadows are always formed on the opposite side of the jaw and at a higher level than the real image, and are variably magnified, particularly in the horizontal plane.

102(a) Magnetic resonance imaging, a useful technique for demonstrating the soft tissues; since it is a non-invasive procedure, it is increasingly used as an alternative to TMJ arthrography (see **5**).

(b) The views show the right TMJ in a sagittal profile in the open and closed positions. In the closed position (**102A**), the disc, which has a low signal intensity and appears as a black biconcave structure, lies anteriorly to the head of the mandibular condyle. In addition, the head of the condyle appears to lie in a more retruded position within the glenoid fossa. *[Note: The cortical bone also has a low signal intensity (black), while the marrow has a high signal intensity (white).]* On opening (**102B**), the disc is situated in a normal position overlying the condylar head.

(c) The condition illustrated is an anterior displacement of the TMJ disc with reduction on opening. In patients with TMJ dysfunction, the 'click' is associated with the sudden movement (reduction) of the disc to a more normal position during the movement of the condylar head on opening.

103(a) There is a periapical radiolucency, approximately 20 mm in diameter, involving the apices of |12 It is trapezoid in shape and its outline is well-defined and largely corticated. The lamina dura around much of the apical portion of |2 is absent. The crown |2 is missing.

(b) The most likely diagnosis is a radicular (periapical) cyst. A periapical radiolucency which has a diameter greater than 20 mm and is associated with a non-vital tooth is more likely to be a periapical cyst than a periapical granuloma.

(c) During root canal preparation, a root canal file has broken within the root canal. In order to facilitate its removal an attempt has been made to drill around the fragment of instrument, resulting in the fracture of the end part of a small round bur, which lies distal to the file.

104	**Radiation Protection Supervisor**	**Radiation Protection Advisor**
Qualifications	Normally a dentist but can be a suitably trained dental nurse: must command sufficient respect from all those working in the practice	Medical physicist or other suitably experienced person who is normally employed by a radiation protection service
Statutory requirements	Must be appointed	A dental practice is exempt from employing a RPA under certain specified conditions (see *Radiation Protection in Dental Practice*, paragraph 1.4, page 6)
Duties	Ensure all staff observe *Local Rules* and comply with *Ionising Radiation Regulations and related Guidance Notes.*	Advise on the observance of the *Ionising Radiation Regulations* and related *Guidance Notes.*

105(a) A circular, unilocular, radiolucent lesion is situated in the mandible, in front of the angle and between the lower border and the inferior alveolar canal. Its margin is well-defined and well-corticated. The inferior alveolar canal appears to deviate in relation to the radiolucency, but otherwise does not appear to be affected.

(b) Stafne's idiopathic bone cavity, a cavity or depression on the lingual aspect of the mandible which occupies a characteristic site at the angle of the mandible and below the inferior alveolar canal. The aetiology is unknown, but several theories have been postulated, including that the cavity contains aberrant salivary gland tissue or that it is caused by pressure atrophy from the facial artery. Although sometimes described as a static bone cavity, there have been reports that show that the defect can increase in size with age. Similarly produced radiolucencies have been reported in relation to the parotid and sublingual salivary glands.

(c) A sialogram of the left submandibular gland may be helpful in confirming the presence of salivary tissue in the cavity. Otherwise no further investigations are usually required, although when doubt remains a computerized tomographic scan may be indicated.

106(a) There is a multiloculated, clearly defined radiolucency located between the roots $\overline{43}$. It has a mostly corticated margin and is separated into distinct locules by bony septae. The roots of both teeth have been displaced away from the lesion.

ANSWERS

(b) The following conditions should be considered in the differential diagnosis:

(i) Odontogenic keratocyst.

(ii) Ameloblastoma.

(iii) Giant cell lesion.

(iv) Botyroid lateral periodontal cyst.

(v) Odontogenic myxoma.

(vi) Glandular odontogenic cyst.

(c) (i) A lower true occlusal radiograph should be taken to assess the extent of the expansion, buccolingually.

(ii) Biopsy – because of its relatively small size and non-malignant radiographic appearance, an excisional biopsy is more appropriate than an incisional one. Aspiration of the lesion may also be attempted prior to excision, to determine whether the lesion is cystic in nature.

This lesion was diagnosed as a botyroid lateral periodontal cyst. Lateral periodontal cysts are developmental in origin, usually unilocular, and relatively uncommon. Occasionally, they may be multilocular, as in this example, when macroscopically the lesion can appear as a bunch of grapes, hence the name botyroid. The site in this example is typical of the condition. The lesion was treated by local excision; careful follow-up is recommended because the multilocularity may predispose to local recurrence.

107(a) There is delayed eruption of most of the teeth of the permanent dentition and retention of many of the primary teeth. Only the first molars and the lower central incisors have erupted. All the permanent teeth have formed, although there is some delay in their development. In addition, there are several supernumerary teeth in the anterior parts of both upper and lower jaws.

(b) Cleidocranial dysplasia, an uncommon developmental disorder which may be transmitted as an autosomal dominant or appear spontaneously; it mainly affects the skull, teeth, and clavicles. Cranial involvement includes:

(i) Delayed closure of the fontanelles.

(ii) Multiple sutures, especially in the occipital region, producing small sutural bones (wormian bones).

(iii) Underdevelopment of the maxilla to produce a relative mandibular prognathism. Dental involvement includes:

(i) Numerous unerupted supernumerary teeth.

(ii) Delayed eruption of the permanent dentition.

(iii) Prolonged retention of the primary dentition.

(iv) Abnormal cementum of the roots of the primary and permanent dentition, which is the probable cause of the delayed eruption of the teeth.

(i) The Clavicles may be partially or completely absent, so that those affected are able to approximate their shoulders in front of the chest.

There may be other ossification defects, notably affecting the pelvis.

(c) Management involves a balance between facilitating the eruption of the permanent dentition, where this is feasible, the maintenance of the remaining primary teeth, and the provision of overdentures.

108(a) Dilaceration of the upper right central incisor – its root is markedly hooked, typical of this condition (dilaceration is a sharp bend or curve of a tooth root). This tooth is unerupted and rotated through 90°, with its labial surface pointing distally. Because 1⌋ was displaced and failed to erupt, 2⌋ has drifted and tilted mesially.

(b) The most likely cause for this abnormality is a traumatic injury to the primary incisor, resulting in this tooth being intruded into the alveolus, so displacing and damaging the developing permanent incisor. Dilaceration of a permanent central incisor usually occurs after its crown has formed, but while its root is still developing. The traumatic event displaces the calcified portion of the tooth more than the soft tissue component of the developing root, leaving them in an abnormal and angled relationship to each other. Thus, the root develops at an angle to the crown, giving a hooked appearance, and it may also be shorter than normal.

Dilaceration may affect teeth other than the upper central incisor, particularly wisdom teeth and premolars. In many instances (including upper central incisors), there is no history of trauma, in which case it is probable that the cause is a developmental anomaly.

(c) In this example, the position and abnormal shape of 1⌋ and the loss of space in the upper left incisor region indicate that 1⌋ should be removed surgically. Subsequently, the crown of 2⌋ may be restored to simulate the appearance of 1⌋. In situations when the dilacerated tooth is not particularly deformed and there is sufficient room to accommodate it within the alveolus, surgical exposure may be appropriate.

(d) The nasolacrimal canal.

109(a) There are fractures of the incisal aspect of the crowns of both teeth. Access cavities have been prepared into the coronal pulp chambers, the outlines of which are rectangular and wider than normal, and are partly filled with a radiopaque material. In the mid-portion of both roots there is a horizontal calcific bridge separating the apical and coronal parts of the root. The apical parts of the roots appear normal and the periapical lamina duras are intact.

(b) As a consequence of the fracture, the pulps of both teeth were exposed. In order to reach the vital, non-inflamed pulp tissue, pulpotomies have been carried out at a more apical level than normal. Following the application of calcium hydroxide dressings, both roots have responded with the formation of calcific bridges and the completion of root development.

(c) As the pulp tissue in the apical parts of the roots remains vital, restoration of only the coronal parts of the teeth may be all that is necessary. Alternatively, penetration of the calcific barriers allowing conventional root-filling treatment and post crown preparations may be required.

110(a) There is a fusiform, uniform radiopacity extending from the mesial aspect of ⌐4 to the distal aspect ⌐5. It is well-defined and its margin merges with that of the adjacent alveolar bone.

(b) Mandibular torus, a developmental bony hyperplasia which is usually bilateral and found on the lingual aspect of the mandible in the premolar region. Mandibular tori are usually diagnosed in adulthood, are asymptomatic, and of variable size. When small they are not usually sufficiently dense to be visible on periapical radiographs. They do not normally require removal unless they interfere with the wearing of a lower denture. The

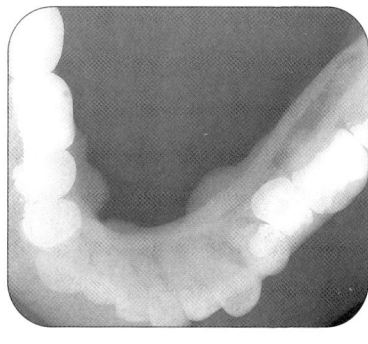

off-set lower true (90°) occlusal radiograph (above) demonstrates the nature of the lesion and also shows a bilobed torus on the right side.

(c) The differential diagnosis as observed on a periapical radiograph includes osteosclerosis, hypercementosis, cemental tumour, and an osteoma.

111(a) The dental panoramic radiograph (**111A**) shows considerable destruction of the bone of the edentulous alveolus from the canine to the tuberosity region in the upper left quadrant of the mouth. The antral floor and part of the outline of the hard palate is missing.

The occipitomental radiograph (**111B**) confirms the bone loss in the lower part of the left maxillary antrum. It also shows that the entire antrum is radiopaque and that there is bone destruction of the lateral wall and roof. However, the orbital rim and the infra-orbital foramen remain intact.

(b) Carcinoma of the maxillary antrum – the clinical features which may be present in this disorder (in addition to pain and swelling) include nasal obstruction, recurrent sinusitis, epistaxis, epiphora, and infra-orbital nerve paraesthesia. As this lesion frequently develops on the floor of the maxillary antrum, dental symptoms may also be a presenting feature. These include expansion or swelling of the alveolus in the molar or premolar region, resulting in difficulty wearing an upper denture. Destruction of the alveolar bone may result in loosening of the upper posterior teeth. Eventually, the tumour may erode through the bone to present as a mass in the oral cavity.

(c) Incisional biopsy of the lesion is essential to establish the diagnosis. Computerized tomographic scanning and/or magnetic resonance imaging are required to determine the extent of the lesion and the presence of lymph node deposits, and thus assist in the choice of treatment options.

112(a) A diagnostic ultrasound image.

(b) High frequency sound waves are transmitted from a transducer, placed upon the surface of the skin, into the underlying soft tissues. A frequency in the region of 7.5 MHz, for example, is used to image the tissues in the region of the jaws. The velocity of sound waves through the tissues varies with their compressibility and density. At the interface of tissues with different sound conduction properties (acoustic impedances), some of the sound waves are reflected back to the transducer where they are received and converted into an electronic signal. The signals are displayed on a television monitor and recorded on film. The remaining sound waves penetrate further into the tissues until their energy is dissipated.

(c) The skin surface is at the top of the illustration, below which is a 'heart'-shaped hypoechoic (dark) area showing no internal structures. Deep to this area is a zone of acoustic enhancement (white area). These features are typical of a cystic or fluid-filled lesion, such as a ranula (as in this example), a dermoid cyst, or possibly an abscess.

113(a) A unilocular, expansive radiolucent lesion is situated in the midline of the mandible between the lower central incisors. The roots of the incisors have both been displaced distally, but there is no evidence of resorption. The inferior margin is smooth, moderately well-defined, but apparently not corticated.

(b) The differential diagnosis includes:
(i) Central giant cell granuloma (the diagnosis in this example), a non-neoplastic lesion that predominantly affects adolescents or young adults. It occurs most commonly in the anterior part of the mandible and may cross the midline. When small, it appears as a cyst-like radiolucency, but larger lesions are typically multilocular and contain bony trabeculae. It tends to cause displacement of the tooth roots (as in this example), rather than root resorption.
(ii) Odontogenic keratocyst.
(iii) Lateral periodontal cyst.
(iv) Brown tumour of hyperparathyroidism, a condition that usually develops in middle age.

(c) Other investigations could include:
(i) A lower true (90°) occlusal radiograph to assess any buccolingual expansion of the mandible.
(ii) Other intra-oral radiographs may be helpful to determine if there are changes in the trabecular pattern elsewhere in the jaws.
(iii) A dental panoramic tomograph to assess whether there are other similar lesions elsewhere in the jaws.
(iv) A serum biochemical profile to assess the levels of calcium, alkaline phosphatase, and parathormone levels, which would be abnormal in hyperparathyroidism.
(v) Aspiration biopsy to determine the presence of fluid.

114(a) There is an oval radiolucency situated in the anterior aspect of the ramus of the mandible on the right side. It extends from the retromolar region to the base of the coronoid process and to within approximately 1 cm of the posterior aspect of the ramus. It is well-defined and partly corticated. Although essentially unilocular, the superior margin is scalloped because of the formation of an incomplete septum. There is thinning and slight expansion of the anterior cortical margin of the mandibular ramus.

(b) Odontogenic keratocyst (which has become infected) – other intra-osseous tumours, notably ameloblastomas, may have a similar radiographic appearance, but rarely become infected and generally are painless. However, infection is a common presenting symptom in patients with odontogenic keratocysts. Typically, odontogenic keratocysts have the following radiographic features:

(i) A unilocular oval radiolucency, often with a scalloped margin.

(ii) They occur most commonly in the molar or retromolar region of the mandible.

(iii) The margins are well-defined and often corticated.

(iv) Large lesions assume an elongated appearance, as they enlarge through the cancellous spaces rather than by expansion of the bony cortical plates. However, thinning of the bony cortex does occur and bony perforations may be noted.

(v) They may develop adjacent to an unerupted tooth, to assume an apparent dentigerous relationship, or to the roots of an erupted tooth to resemble a lateral periodontal cyst. Tooth displacement is common; however, root resorption is not.

(vi) Maxillary lesions can occupy much or all of the antrum.

(vii) Computerized tomography is helpful in demonstrating the presence of bony perforation and the relationship between the cyst and the maxillary antrum.

(viii) They are usually solitary, but sometimes multiple, in which case naevoid basal cell carcinoma syndrome should be suspected.

115(a) Dental panoramic tomographs (TMJ programme view), taken with the mouth open.

(b) There is a small erosion of part of the articular surface of the right mandibular condyle. The left condyle head is flattened and there is a linear margin of sclerosis affecting the articular surface and anterior condylar aspect.

(c) Osteoarthrosis of the TMJ.

(d) Osteoarthrosis of the TMJ is a common degenerative condition, which may be seen in the second or third decades of life, but is frequently found in middle-aged or elderly patients, when it tends to be asymptomatic. Clinical features of this condition are pain and tenderness of the affected joints (particularly when eating chewy foods), joint crepitus, and limitation of mandibular opening.

(e) Radiographic features (other than erosion and sclerosis) include osteophyte formation, disk displacement, and disk perforation. The condylar head usually undergoes gradual remodelling to assume a flattened appearance. Sclerosis of the glenoid fossa and flattening of the articular eminence often occur at the same time as the condylar changes.

116(a) There are two focal collections of radiopacities, one lying postero-inferiorly to the left angle of the mandible and the other lying more inferiorly. Both groups consist of several discrete radiopacities of varying size, shape, and density; the larger ones having lobulated outlines.

(b) Dystrophic mineralization of cervical lymph nodes, probably as a consequence of previous infection with *Mycobacterium tuberculosis*. Radiographically, such lymph nodes have an appearance described typically as resembling a cauliflower. Compare the appearance and position of these soft tissue calcifications with those of the mineralized salivary gland illustrated in **34**.

110

(c) The linear radiopaque lines are ghost or secondary images produced on the opposite side of the radiograph by the calcified lymph nodes.

117(a) The anterior teeth are magnified ('stretched out') in a horizontal direction and appear blurred. In addition, the secondary shadows (ghost images) of the mandible are prominent on both sides and a 'streak artefact' (secondary shadow of a dental restoration) overlies the left maxillary canine and premolars. All these features are a consequence of the patient being positioned too far posteriorly relative to the focal plane, and with the chin up.

(b) Extreme care must be taken to ensure that the teeth and jaws lie within the focal plane of the tomograph. In this correct position, horizontal and vertical magnification on the radiograph are the same (around 30%). The image of any structure lying lateral (buccal) to the focal plane will show proportionally less horizontal magnification. In contrast, any structure medial (lingual) to the focal plane will exhibit proportionally excessive horizontal distortions. In the example illustrated, the anteroposterior head position was incorrect, with the patient's head being placed too far posteriorly relative to the focal plane. Thus, the anterior teeth appear magnified and poorly defined.

Modern panoramic equipment incorporates aids to positioning, such as light beams, bite blocks, chin rests, forehead rests, and cephalostats. The best way to avoid the type of error illustrated here is to follow carefully the manufacturer's instructions concerning positioning.

118 The spacer cone contains a rectangular collimator. In this example the collimator has been designed to reduce the dimensions of the beam at the cone tip from a diameter of 6 cm to a rectangle measuring to 4.5×3.5 cm, equivalent to a Size 2 dental X-ray film. Rectangular collimation has two advantages: there is a 40% reduction in patient-absorbed dose (and a similar reduction in scattered radiation to the operator) and image contrast is improved due to the decrease in scattered radiation. On the other hand, correct beam alignment is more difficult and the use of beam-aligning devices is therefore essential.

119(a) Tunnel restorations – the one on the upper left premolar has been performed through an existing occlusal amalgam restoration.

(b) Two different materials have been used to restore the cavities. A radiolucent glass ionomer cement [Chemfil] was used to fill the upper right premolar and a radiopaque cement [Ketac Silver] the upper left premolar. A radiopaque material makes the recognition of the restoration and the diagnosis of recurrent caries easier. A radiolucent restorative material may resemble dental caries, as in this example.

120(a) His appearance, as he has dentinogenesis imperfecta and the teeth usually have an opalescent bluish-brown colour. Occasionally, dentinogenesis imperfecta is associated with osteogenesis imperfecta, in which case the patient may also have blue sclera.

(b) The primary dentition has suffered extensively from attrition and most of the enamel has been lost. The permanent teeth have somewhat bulbous crowns, with relatively short roots. The coronal pulp chambers are already partially obliterated, particularly in the erupted teeth.

(c) Histologically, the enamel is likely to be normal, although in approximately one-third of those affected with dentinogenesis imperfecta there are areas of hypomineralization. The ameledentinal junction is described classically as flattened and lacking the normal scalloped appearance. The mantle dentine is relatively normal, but the circumpulpal dentine has a poorly mineralized matrix with numerous areas of interglobular dentine. There may be abnormal whorled areas of dentine matrix and cellular inclusions. The dentinal tubules are fewer in number and more irregular in orientation and distribution than in normal teeth. Pulpal necrosis is commonly present, as a consequence of the rapid attrition.

121(a) A well-defined, multilocular lesion extends from the lower left canine to the lower left second molar. Its full extent cannot be determined from this view. The lesion consists of numerous small round lobules, giving a soap bubble or honeycombed appearance. There is extensive resorption of both roots of the lower first molar, as well as some resorption of the premolars.

(b) The radiographic differential diagnosis of an aggressive multilocular lesion in this age group includes ameloblastoma (as in this example) and myxoma. Ameloblastoma is a benign, but locally invasive, neoplasm of odontogenic epithelium which occurs in two main histological forms, follicular and plexiform. The follicular type more commonly causes a honeycomb pattern of bone destruction, whereas the plexiform type is more often associated with cystic radiolucencies (see **1**). Both types often cause root resorption and, when marked, this is an important diagnostic feature. Odontogenic myxoma, which is a benign neoplasm of odontogenic mesenchyme, may cause a similar radiographic appearance. The internal septa within the myxoma are said to be finer and straighter than those in the ameloblastoma, and are therefore sometimes described as resembling the strings of a tennis racket.

122(a) Upper oblique occlusal radiograph centred on 3̲2̲|(**122A**) and an upper anterior (standard) occlusal radiograph (**122B**).

(b) 3̲| lies in a buccal position relative to the upper incisor teeth, as determined by the principle of parallax. In the first view (**122A**), the crown of 3̲| is superimposed upon the root of 2̲| as far as its mesial aspect. In the second view (**122B**), the crown of 3̲|appears to be in a more distal position, only reaching as far as the root canal of 2̲|. That is, as the tube has moved in a mesial direction from (**122A**) to (**122B**), the crown of 3̲|appears to have moved in the opposite (distal) direction.

123(a) There is moderate, horizontal bone loss of the alveolar crest affecting |4̄5̄6̄7̄, with early involvement of the bifurcation |6̄. Associated with the distal root |6̄, there is a localized area of bone destruction which extends down to the apex. This defect involves only one of the cortical plates (buccal or lingual), as the shadow of the other is visible at the apical half of the distal root. In addition there is widening of the periodontal ligament along the mesial surface of the distal root ⎾6. Large coronal restorations are present in ⏋567, and there is some sclerosis of the mesial root canal⎾6.

(b) Chronic adult periodontitis with localized extension on the distal root ⎾6 to produce a periodontal–endodontic lesion.

(c) Treatment options include:
  (i) Extraction.
  (ii) Root canal therapy followed by periodontal scaling and root planing, with or without guided tissue regeneration.
  (iii) Root canal therapy followed by root resection of the distal root.
  (iv) Root canal therapy followed by hemisection and subsequent crowning of the remaining tooth tissue to appear as a premolar, which was the option adopted in this case.

124(a) There is a clearly defined oval radiolucency measuring approximately 3×5 mm, separated a short distance from the apex of ⎿2 by a bridge of normal bone. The tooth is root-filled and contains an obliquely inclined gold post, and the flattened apex contains a retrograde amalgam filling. The periodontal ligament space and the lamina dura appear normal. There is healthy bone between the root apex and the radiolucent area.

(b) A fibrous scar following the apical surgery; these occur as the result of incomplete bony regeneration, usually involving one or both cortical plates, and thus causing a radiolucent 'punched out' appearance. Scar formation is more likely to occur if there is damage to the periosteum at the time of surgery. If the radiolucency is projected upon the apex of a tooth it may simulate a periapical inflammatory lesion.

(c) No treatment is necessary, as fibrous scars are asymptomatic and may slowly reduce in size with time. If the diagnosis is in doubt, a further radiograph taken 1 year later may help to confirm it.

125(a) A reduced exposure submentovertex radiograph (jug-handle view).

(b) There is a depressed fracture of the right zygomatic arch with medial (inwards) displacement of the bone fragments.

(c) The cardinal signs and symptoms include deformity of the facial outline overlying the zygomatic arch, limitation of opening of the mouth, and facial pain.

(d) Fracture reduction would be necessary in the presence of an altered facial appearance and/or limitation of opening of the mouth. The fracture is treated by elevation of the depressed fragments using a Gillie's temporal approach. Fixation of the reduced fragments may be necessary if they remain unstable.

126(a) There is displacement of the left malar bone with a fracture through the zygomatic arch and separation of the bones at the frontozygomatic suture. There is also a comminuted fracture through the left infra-orbital margin in the region of the infra-orbital foramen. The lateral wall of the left maxillary antrum is buckled. The diastema between the upper central incisor teeth is natural.

(b) The patient's symptoms and clinical signs might include:
  (i) Pain, swelling, and bruising over the left cheek and around the left eye.
  (ii) Flattening of the face on the left.
  (iii) Subconjunctival haemorrhage in the left eye.
  (iv) Numbness over the left cheek and of the teeth in the upper left quadrant.
  (v) Diplopia.
  (vi) Restricted movement of the globe of the left eye.
  (vii) Inequality of the pupillary levels.
  (viii) Bruising and tenderness in the buccal sulcus.
  (ix) Slight alteration in the occlusion.
(c) The most important further investigation relates to assessing the shape and continuity of the bone around the left orbit. In particular, the possibility of orbital floor damage must be evaluated, for which computerized tomographic scanning would be appropriate.

127(a) The radiograph shows $\overline{678}$. There is widening of the periodontal ligament space apically on the mesial root $\overline{7}$, together with a zone of radiopacity, indicative of sclerosing osteitis from chronic irritation. The wisdom tooth is mesio-angularly impacted against $\overline{7}$. The follicular space distally $\overline{8}$ is enlarged, probably due to recurrent episodes of pericoronitis. Thus, either $\overline{7}$ or $\overline{8}$ are possible causes of the patient's complaint.
(b) From the evidence presented in the radiograph, the cause of the discomfort is uncertain. It would be preferable, therefore, to investigate the condition of the pulp of $\overline{7}$ and undertake the appropriate conservation of this tooth, rather than remove the impacted wisdom tooth, particularly because its roots are probably grooved by the inferior alveolar canal. This latter feature is apparent as there is an abrupt alteration of the radiodensity of the mesial root, which is less dense where it is crossed by the canal. In addition, there is a slight narrowing and sudden change of direction of the canal at this point, and the cortical lamina of the canal appears deficient as it crosses the root of $\overline{8}$. Thus, the removal of the wisdom tooth is likely to result in damage to the inferior alveolar nerve. Should the discomfort persist, extraction of either or both teeth may be necessary. If $\overline{8}$ requires removal, it would be advisable to refer the patient to a specialist oral surgeon.

128(a) A vertex occlusal radiograph.
(b) A cassette, containing screen film and intensifying screens, is protected from the oral environment by a plastic bag and inserted into the mouth against the occlusal surfaces of the maxillary teeth. The X-ray cone is placed on the vertex of the head and the tube angled so that the central X-ray beam passes down the long axis of the upper central incisor teeth. This radiograph demonstrates the upper anterior teeth in plan view. N.B. It is essential that the patient wears a lead apron.
(c) There is a palatally displaced unerupted upper left canine. Its crown lies close to the left incisor teeth and the root is curved apically. The upper left primary canine is retained. The circular radiolucency overlying the root of the $\underline{3}$ is the nasolacrimal canal.

(d) (i) Less sharpness compared with that obtained with direct exposure film, because of the need to use screen film and intensifying screens.

(ii) Superimposition of the images of the dense bones of the facial skeleton upon the anterior teeth.

(iii) Irradiation of much of the body because of the downwards angulation of the X-ray beam.

(iv) The relatively great distance between the X-ray tube and the maxillary teeth adds to the difficulty of precision in beam alignment. The anterior teeth must be demonstrated in plan view when assessing the buccopalatal position of an unerupted tooth in the anterior part of the maxilla.

129(a) There is a unilocular, radiolucent lesion, approximately 3 cm in diameter, in the $\overline{67}$ region of the mandible. It has a slightly scalloped margin, which is well-defined, but not obviously corticated, and appears punched out of the bone. The bone of the alveolar crest is perforated above, where there is a smooth soft-tissue swelling. There is no evidence of calcification within the lesion.

(b) Radiographic differential diagnosis includes:

(i) Eosinophilic granuloma.

(ii) A lesion of multiple myeloma (see also **97**).

(iii) Central fibroma.

(iv) Odontogenic keratocyst.

Histology showed the lesion to be an eosinophilic granuloma, a form of Langerhan's cell histiocytosis (histiocytosis X), which occurs in three different clinical patterns, namely:

(i) Solitary eosinophilic granuloma (as in this case).

(ii) Multifocal eosinophilic granuloma (Hands–Schüller–Christian disease)

(iii) Letterer–Siwe disease.

In all three conditions the bone lesions are similar and are caused by a proliferation of Langerhan's cells and eosinophilic leucocytes. Typically, they appear punched out and, when they occur in the tooth-bearing portion of the jaws, may cause marked destruction of the alveolar bone (without causing root resorption), so that the teeth appear radiographically to be floating or standing in space. Treatment varies according to the clinical form of the disease.

130(a) A true lateral view of the anterior maxilla with a reduced exposure to demonstrate the soft tissues. It is usually taken on an occlusal film using a dental X-ray set.

(b) There is a radiopaque fragment from the crown of an upper tooth (probably an incisor) present within the substance of the upper lip, which is swollen. The fragment has rotated so that its labial and palatal surfaces lie at right angles to the surface of the lip.

131(a) The outline of the tooth is abnormal, with the crown appearing conical in shape and the root wider than normal (dilated). Also, the tooth is rotated. Arising from the lingual aspect of the crown is an invagination of mineralized dental tissues which is lined by a thin layer of densely radiopaque enamel and reaches to the apical third of the root. The displaced radiolucent pulp chamber is narrow and can be seen pushed back to each side of the invagination. There is a periapical radiolucency with loss of lamina dura, the full extent of which is not recorded on this radiograph. In addition there is a well-defined radiolucency in the distal part of the crown.

(b) Invaginated odontome (dens in dente). Since these invaginations are usually incompletely protected by enamel, pulpal infection and necrosis commonly occurs, leading subsequently to periapical inflammation, as is illustrated in this example.

(c) There is a punched out, clearly defined radiolucency, overlying most of the crown of the tooth. This appearance is typical of a carious lesion occurring on the buccal or lingual surface of the crown. There is a similar lesion in the crown of 2|.

132(a) External root resorption, there being two apparently separate areas of resorption, one distally and one overlying the root canal, both in the coronal aspect of the root.

(b) The necrotic pulp should have been extirpated from the tooth some 7–10 days after reimplantation. Following mechanical preparation and debridement of the canal, a non-setting calcium hydroxide dressing should have been inserted into the root canal to minimize the possibility of root resorption.

(c) The most important prognostic factors are:
(i) The conditions under which the tooth was stored following avulsion.
(ii) The length of time between avulsion and reimplantation.
(iii) The integrity of the socket wall and the tooth.
(iv) Adequate splinting following reimplantation.
(v) The provision of prophylactic antibiotics immediately following reimplantation.

133(a) This diagram shows the photoelectric effect (photoelectric absorption) in which an X-ray photon is absorbed completely by an atom, resulting in the ejection of a photo-electron from its orbit (usually the inner K shell). The loss of an electron converts the atom into a positive ion (ionization). The rearrangements of the remaining electrons causes the emission of characteristic radiation. This is of such low energy that it is absorbed within the patient and does not fog the film. The ejected photo-electron interacts with other atoms until its energy is dissipated.

(b) The frequency of photo-electric absorption is directly proportional to the third power of the atomic number of the constituents of the absorbing material; thus, more photoelectric interactions will occur in bone (higher atomic number) than in water. Such interactions occur predominantly at low beam energies, leading to a relatively higher contrast scale.

134(a) The film is generally dark with low contrast; even the image of the amalgam restoration in the lower molar is grey, rather than densely radiopaque. This appearance is described as 'fogging'.

(b) There are a number of causes, including:
(i) The use of time-expired film.
(ii) The use of incorrectly stored film, for example:

- Environment too hot.
- Too close to an X-ray source without appropriate protection.

(iii) Light fogging might arise, for example, if:
- A box of films was inadvertently exposed by forgetting to replace the lid.
- A cassette is not light-proof.
- The darkroom is not light-tight or has an inappropriate safe-light.

(iv) Chemical fogging might arise from the use of developer, for example:
- At an excessively high temperature.
- For a prolonged period of time.
- At too great a concentration.

(c) Check the following:

(i) The film stock, noting the 'use by' date and the storage conditions.

(ii) The film batch is not fogged by processing an unexposed film from the same box.

(iii) The temperature and concentration of the developer solution.

(iv) The darkroom procedure used by the person who processed the film.

(v) The light-tightness of the darkroom, which can be done simply by standing in the darkroom with the door closed and the lights off and looking for light leaks.

(vi) The darkroom safe-lights, for which the bulb should not exceed 25 W, the filter should match the manufacturer's recommendation and should not be damaged, and the light should be no closer than 1.2 m from where the films are handled. Perform a standard coin test.

135(a) There is an enlarged follicular space around the crown of the unerupted $\overline{7|}$, within which are two small relatively dense, discrete radiopacities, one mesio-occlusally and the other disto-occlusally. $\overline{7|}$ is displaced distally, slightly more than would be expected relative to the size of the lesion, which also appears to have prevented $\overline{7|}$ from erupting. $\overline{8|}$ is congenitally absent.

(b) Ameloblastic fibro-odontome, developing compound odontome, and calcifying epithelial odontogenic tumour.

This example was an ameloblastic fibro-odontome, which most commonly develops during the early part of the second decade of life, is usually found in the posterior region of the jaws and is frequently associated with an unerupted tooth. It appears as a well-defined radiolucency containing radiopaque masses distributed throughout the lesion, ranging from a few millimetres up to a centimetre in diameter and sometimes resembling small teeth (denticles). Although the ameloblastic fibro-odontome enlarges slowly it may reach a considerable size. Treatment is surgical enucleation.

136(a) All three root canals contain gutta percha fillings. The mesiobuccal root, which has fractured longitudinally with displacement of the distal fragment, is associated with a well-defined periapical radiolucency, with loss of lamina dura. There is slight elevation of the cortical outline of the floor of the antrum. There is also a poorly defined periapical radiolucency associated with the palatal root and widening of the periodontal ligament space around the distobuccal root. The trifurcation is also radiolucent, indicating bone loss in this area. In this example, the fracture probably occurred from use of excessive force during lateral condensation of the gutta percha.

(b) Extraction of the tooth, after its separation from the bridge, because the prognosis for this tooth is poor. However, as the tooth forms part of the bridge and is the last standing molar, mesiobuccal root resection might be attempted, provided that the other teeth supporting the bridge have a good prognosis. Retreatment of the palatal root canal would also be required.

137 (a) A lower true (90°) occlusal radiograph centred over the lower left premolar and molar region.

(b) Opposite the lower left premolar and first molar teeth, radiopaque striations can be seen beyond the buccal cortex of the mandible, extending perpendicularly for approximately 3–4 mm into the soft tissues. This appearance has been described as sun-ray spiculation and indicates extracortical, subperiosteal, new bone formation. This is due to the shedding of periosteal osteoblasts behind a rapidly growing tumour front, from a neoplasm that has arisen from within the bone.

(c) This appearance is characteristic of an osteosarcoma. However, it may also be a feature of myeloma, osteoblastic metastases, chondrosarcoma, malignant lymphoma, neuroblastoma, advanced cases of Ewing's sarcoma, tuberculosis, and syphilis. Osteosarcomas have ill-defined margins and, according to the proportion of mineralization within the tumours, may appear as radiolucent or radiopaque lesions of variable density. An important early radiological feature is widening, sometimes irregular, of the periodontal ligament space of those teeth involved with the tumour. This appearance should not be confused with chronic periodontal disease.

(d) The socket of the lower left second molar can be identified, but has ill-defined margins and swelling of the overlying soft tissue, both lingually and buccally. These features suggest either acute inflammation of the bone and surrounding tissues or destruction of bone from spread of a malignant tumour.

138 (a) There is a lesion of mixed radiodensity, although it is predominantly radiopaque, occupying the body of the mandible in the $\overline{765}$ region and extending to the lower border. It is well-defined and has a narrow radiolucent periphery, which is clearly depicted except superiorly. The lesion has displaced the inferior alveolar canal inferiorly and the distal root of $\overline{6}$ is markedly resorbed.

(b) Benign cementoblastoma, a rare benign neoplasm of cementum which, unlike the periapical cemental dysplasia, has no racial predilection, usually occurs as a solitary lesion, and is most often diagnosed during the second or third decades of life. It occurs more frequently in men than in women, and is most frequently associated with the lower first permanent molar root. Presenting signs and symptoms include expansion of the mandible and discomfort, which tends to be of low intensity and intermittent in nature. Its radiodensity is variable, depending on its stage of development and the amount of mineral content.

(c) The lesion should be removed as it shows continued growth and may give rise to a pathological fracture. Recurrence is uncommon.

139(a) The radiopacities are caused by substantial deposits of mainly supragingival calculus. Radiopaque spurs of calculus are also visible interstitially on $\overline{345}$. There is moderate horizontal bone loss due to chronic adult periodontitis.

(b) 'The mental foramen', has a 'C' shaped outline and the mental canal is just visible. The radiolucency should not be confused with a periapical inflammatory lesion. The lower second premolar is not carious and the lamina dura around the apex is continuous.

140(a) Hypercementosis, the excessive deposition of cementum upon the external root surface, especially of the apical part of the root. The root has become bulbous and the periodontal ligament space and the lamina dura follow the new root outline. Hypercementosis also affects $\overline{4|}$.

(b) Hypercementosis is usually associated with chronic inflammation, such as in periodontal or periapical disease; however, sometimes there is no obvious cause.

(c) Paget's disease of bone and acromegaly.

141(a) There are fractures of both condylar necks of the mandible. The condylar heads have been displaced by the lateral pterygoid muscles. Such fractures are not uncommon in this type of incident.

(b) In patients with bilateral fractures with displacement of the condylar heads, the occlusion is often deranged with posterior gagging and an anterior open bite. In addition, tooth fractures may occur. In this radiograph, the restoration in the upper left first molar is missing, possibly as a consequence of the trauma. The retaining pin is still present distally and there is a periapical radiolucency.

(c) A view, at right angles to the dental panoramic tomograph, of the postero-anterior condyles to demonstrate their displacement in a mediolateral plane. This information may also be obtained from a Towne's (or reverse Towne's) radiograph.

142(a) There is a densely radiopaque 'bowler-hat'-shaped metallic foreign body overlying the body of the mandible in the molar region. Several smaller, less dense particles are present anterior to the main fragment.

(b) A true lateral radiograph of the mandible and a lower true (90°) occlusal radiograph, i.e., views at right angles to the one illustrated, would be necessary to demonstrate the spatial relationship and the exact position of the foreign bodies relative to the mandible.

(c) An air gun pellet which has lodged against the lateral aspect of the mandible. The shape of the main portion of the pellet has been distorted upon impact with the

bone. Its trajectory through the soft tissue is demonstrated by the distribution of the smaller fragments.

(d) Low velocity bullets carry a risk of infection and should be removed, wherever possible. In addition, appropriate antibiotic therapy and antitetanus prophylaxis should be carried out. In this case, the air gun pellet was palpable in the buccal sulcus and was removed under general anaesthesia via an intra-oral approach. It is advisable to keep the removed fragments for mediolegal reference.

143 The patient was positioned with the head tilted too far inferiorly, so that the coronoid and condylar processes of the mandible and much of the maxilla lie above the upper margin of the film. In addition, the patient's neck was curved anteriorly so that the X-ray beam passed through more of the cervical spine than if the neck had been straight, resulting in a prominent radiopaque midline shadow. The film lacks density, because of either underexposure or underdevelopment.

144(a) (i) There is a roughly circular, well-defined radiolucency, approximately 10 mm in diameter, involving the apices of 31| and extending up to the floor of the nose. The lamina dura around the apical aspect of both teeth is missing. Contained within the root canal of 1| is some radiopaque material.
(ii) Absence of the right upper lateral incisor: in this patient it was congenitally missing.
(iii) Abnormal morphology of both the crown and root of the right upper canine. The crown appears invaginated (invaginated odontome) and there is an accessory root canal due to the presence of the invaginated odontome on the mesial aspect.
(b) Conventional root canal therapy to 31|; however, this may be difficult due to the irregularity of the pulp chamber and the abnormal root canal morphology of the canine. Ultrasonic instrumentation may facilitate mechanical preparation of the root canal. Obturation of the accessory root canal would also be necessary. In view of the size of the periapical radiolucency, radiographic follow up is advisable. If the periapical inflammatory lesion fails to resolve following root canal therapy, apical surgery should be considered.

145(a) A cross-sectional tomographic slice taken vertically through the right side of the body of the mandible in the premolar region. This type of tomographic slice of the jaws can be produced by recently developed multidirectional tomographic machines, such as the Scanora® or Tomax Ultrascan®.
(b) The body of the mandible is expanded both buccally and lingually, particularly in the inferior aspect. Much of the bone appears to have a ground-glass appearance, although on the buccal aspect there are several discrete radiolucencies. Lingually, the cortical margin is sclerotic and there are several radiopaque foci inferolaterally. The cortical bone appears to be intact all round the lesion (compare this example with **41**). The crowns of the teeth, at the top of the illustration, appear blurred as they are adjacent to, but not in the plane of, this tomograph.
(c) This is a benign expansile lesion throughout which there are areas of mineralization of varying density; the most likely diagnosis is a cemento-ossifying fibroma.

146(a) Systemic sclerosis.
(b) This is a rare connective tissue disorder diagnosed mainly in middle-aged women and resulting in fibrosis of the subcutaneous tissues and viscera, including the

gastrointestinal tract, heart, lungs, and kidneys. Initially, the hands are affected by Raynaud's phenomenon and by painful joints. Involvement of the skin leads to a claw-like deformity of the hands and tautness of the face, resulting in restricted mouth opening and a mask-like facial appearance. A characteristic dental radiological feature is widening of the periodontal ligament space which is found in over 10% of cases. Bone resorption, often bilateral, may occur at the sites of muscle attachment to the jaws, typically the angle of the mandible, the coronoid process, and the zygomatic arch.

(c) Other causes of widening of the periodontal ligament space include:
(i) Periapical inflammation.
(ii) Periodontal inflammation.
(iii) Occlusal traumatism.
(iv) Tooth subluxation.
(v) A fracture involving a tooth socket.
(vi) A radiographic projection effect.
(vii) Osteogenic sarcoma.
(viii) Burkitt's lymphoma.
The widening may be confined to one or several adjacent teeth (e.g., subluxation, osteogenic sarcoma) or occur in more than one quadrant (e.g., systemic sclerosis and Burkitt's lymphoma).

147(a) **a**, Collimator; **b**, electrostatic focusing cup; **c**, target; **d**, anode; **e**, aluminium filter.
(b) The target consists of tungsten embedded in a copper stem. Tungsten is used because it has a high atomic number (more efficient X-ray production), high melting point (99% of electron kinetic energy is converted into heat), and low vapour pressure, minimizing the contamination of the vacuum in the X-ray tube. On the other hand, tungsten has a relatively low thermal conductivity, in contrast to copper, which has the advantage of high thermal conductivity, so facilitating the dispersal of heat generated at the tungsten target.
(c) Increasing the kilovoltage results in an increased acceleration of the electrons across the X-ray tube and so the conversion of their kinetic energy into X-ray photons. Consequently, there is an increase in:
(i) The mean energy of the photons.
(ii) The maximum energy of the photons.
An increase in the energy of the photons produces an increase in the penetration of the X-ray beam. For example, increasing the kilovoltage peak from 50 to 70 kV decreases the skin surface entrance dose, while increasing the absorbed dose to the deeper tissues. Above 70 kV, changing the kilovoltage has little effect on the absorbed dose. Another effect of increasing the kilovoltage is that the resultant image shows less contrast (appears less black and white) but has a greater range of intermediate shades of grey.

148(a) Interstitial cemental caries – this patient has advanced horizontal periodontal bone loss particularly affecting $\overline{1\,2}$. The bone recession has resulted in exposure of the cemental surfaces of $\overline{1\,2}$, which have developed carious lesions. In contrast to

121

enamel caries, root caries are more broadly based on the surface, as cementum is more rapidly broken down in a similar fashion to that of the underlying dentine. Interstitial root caries may resemble root resorption radiographically (see **27**), but in the former the outline of the lesion is usually less well-defined.

(b) The linear radiolucent lines are due to the presence of intra-osseous vascular channels. They are usually seen on periapical radiographs, most often in the lower incisor and premolar regions. Vascular channels may occur as a normal anatomical feature, but they are more frequently seen in the older patient, in those who have raised blood pressure, and in patients with advanced chronic adult periodontal disease, as in the example illustrated.

149 (a) The lower right wisdom tooth is vertically impacted against the crown of $\overline{7|}$, just below its contact point. The crown of $\overline{8|}$, which is not carious, lies at a slightly lower occlusal level than that of $\overline{7|}$. The wisdom tooth has three roots, two mesially and one distally. The mesial roots are hooked in a distal direction at the apical one-third, while the distal root is straight. The inferior alveolar canal lies immediately beneath the mesial root, but it appears to cross the apex of the distal root, which is more radiolucent than the remainder of the root above the canal. The bony lamina of the roof of the canal appears discontinuous as it crosses the distal root apex **8**, suggesting that the distal root is grooved by the canal. The alveolar crest level lies at the enamel–cement junction mesially, but distally it is at the level of the cusps of the crown. The bone density is normal and the distal follicular space is not enlarged. There is no abnormality of the other teeth.

(b) From the appearance illustrated, it is possible that the distal root apex is grooved by the inferior alveolar canal. If there is a clinical indication to remove the wisdom tooth, another periapical radiograph with a different vertical tube angulation is required. If the shadow of the canal occupies a different position relative to the root it must lie in a different plane to that of the root (principle of parallax). The greater the amount of movement, the further apart the two structures lie.

150 There are numerous restorations and carious lesions indicating that this patient is caries prone. Amalgam restorations are present on $\underline{7654|}$ and $\overline{74|}$, and there is an excess of amalgam at the cervical margin of the filling in $\underline{4|}$. Small, mainly enamel, carious lesions are present on $\underline{7|}$ mesially, distally $\underline{6|}$ distally, $\overline{87|}$ mesially, and a large lesion, extending well into the dentine disto-occlusally on $\overline{5|}$. The lower right first molar is missing and was presumably extracted because of advanced caries a few years after its eruption, allowing $\overline{5|}$ to drift distally and rotate through 90°, so that its lingual surface contacts the mesial aspect of $\overline{7|}$.

INDEX